THE BRAIN & BELIEF

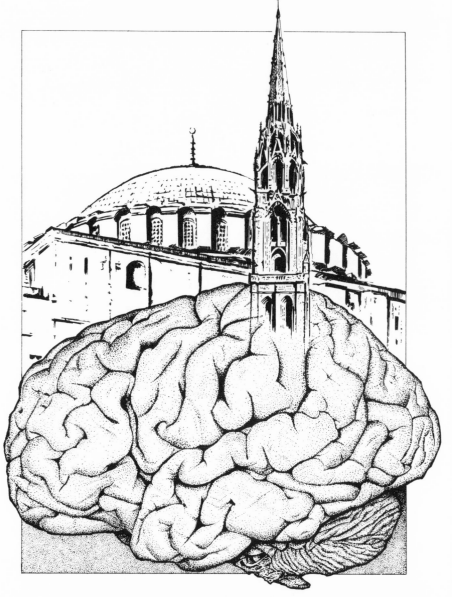

JAMES B. ASHBROOK

THE BRAIN AND BELIEF
Faith in the Light of Brain Research

by

James B. Ashbrook

Library of Congress Catalog Card Number
88-040340

ISBN 1-55605-040-2 (softback)
ISBN 1-55605-041-0 (hardback)

To Pat

whose life is love

whose love is life . . .

ACKNOWLEDGEMENTS

I have been working on "the brain and belief" since the early 1970s. So many individuals have helped I can not begin to name them. Some directed me to special research; others opened doors I might not otherwise have entered; still others challenged, encouraged, and built on my efforts.

Here I mention two: Philip Hefner and Ralph Wendell Burhoe, co-directors of the Chicago Advanced Seminar on Religion In An Age of Science held each spring at the Lutheran School of Theology at Chicago. They have invited me to participate in that forum in numerous ways, ways which have stimulated my thinking, challenged my ideas, and required me to grow. Ralph has been meticulous in scrutinizing my ideas and encouraging that contribution to helping religion be credible in our scientific world. Although his predilection is for the natural sciences and mine for the social sciences, I have found in him -- and his gracious wife Calla -- kindred spirits.

Garrett-Evangelical Theological Seminary could not have been more supportive. Faculty colleagues linked their research with my work; students carried these ideas into areas I would not have imagined; administrators kept insisting my work required the time I was devoting to it. A sabbatical in the fall of 1986 provided psychic space for the difficult task of making its theological and philosophical foundations more explicit. I want to express appreciation to Dean Franklin Sherman for arranging for me to be a Visiting Scholar at the Lutheran School during that period. A sabbatical lecture on the topic "Can The Brain Speak of God?" resulted. In the most tangible way of all, Joan Svenningsen, administrative assistant of the Field of Pastoral Psychology and Counseling, worked with me, my scribbling, our computers, and my uncertainty to translate this material into print. Without her -- her enthusiasm, eagerness, and expertise -- who knows whether the book would have made it.

Barbara Stinchcombe labored with me as an editorial consultant. I say "labored" because labor it was. She managed to reshape my convoluted writing into a semblance of clarity, thereby making its contribution accessible in a way not otherwise possible. She is a free lance editor who also works as an editorial assistant with the Dissertation Office at The University of Chicago, as well as her being a poetress in her own right. She helped me find my "voice" and shared her "voice."

Keith McBarron is an exquisite illustrator. He designed the cover, drew the four illustrations -- actually works of art -- of St. Sophia and Chartres Cathedral, and executed the two figures which integrate brain processes and patterns of belief. The cover is stunning, as publisher John Morgan knew it would be when he engaged Keith to do the art work.

John Morgan, publisher of Wyndham Hall Press and president of The Graduate Theological Foundation, has become a colleague, a friend, and most especially an advocate in making my ideas available to others. We agreed on this project at a special time in my life. I had just learned I was suffering with a recurrence of lymphoma. John's enthusiasm about my work gave me renewed energy in my learning to live with this message from my body about too much uncontrolled growth and overworking my internal vacuum cleaner.

I was privileged to give The Bailey Lectures, 1988, at the American Baptist Seminary of The West in Berkeley, California. For that occasion I used material on architecture (Chapter One), gender (Chapter Two), and pentecostal presence (Chapter Nine). Acting President Theodore Keaton and Acting Dean Benoni Silva-Netto were most generous in their hospitality.

Numerous adult church school classes, pastoral counseling forums, and pastors' workshops have honed these ideas even as the engagements have encouraged me to work with the brain as a resource for belief. Parts of the material on evolution in Chapter Four and epistemology in Chapter Five were used in a presentation to the Science and Theology Section of the American Academy of Religion at its annual convention in Boston in December 1987, under the title "From Being to Brain: Natural Theology in an Empirical Mode."

Paul Rademacher assisted with the original Glossary for Theology, as did J. David Pierce with the Glossary for The Brain with meticulous care. Jane B. Shapley read the final manuscript for accuracy and clarity.

Our grown children Peter, Susan, Martha, and Karen each have played unique roles in the development of these ideas. Their lives and their love mean more to me than I can express. Most of all, my wife Pat, and their mother, has so shared my life that who I am and what she has given are difficult to distinguish. I dedicate this to her -- with words of gratitude and awe.

I am grateful to acknowledge the following:

Excerpts from THE JERUSALEM BIBLE, copyright (c) 1966 by Darton, Longman & Todd, Ltd. and Doubleday, a division of Bantam, Doubleday, Dell Publishing Group, Inc. Reprinted by permission.

Scripture quotations from the Revised Standard Version of the Bible, copyrighted 1946, 1952, 1971 by the Division of Education and Ministry of the National Council of the Churches of Christ in the U.S.A., and used by permission.

Reprinted from Augustine: *Confessions and Enchiridon,* translated and edited by Albert C. Outler (Vol. VII: The Library of Christian Classics). First published MCMLV. Great Britain: SCM, Ltd., London and U.S.A.: The Westminster Press, 1955. Reprinted and used by permission.

From THE HUMAN MIND AND THE MIND OF GOD: Theological Promise in Brain Research (Landham, MD: University Press of America, 1984) and used with permission: Figure 1 Brain, Dome, Spire, page xiii; the following tables with modified and updated information: 2. Theological Contrasts with Suggested Activity of God, page 17; 3. Major Features of the Working Brain, page 45; 4. Features of the Sensory Systems, page 54; 5. Functioning Mind States, page 86; and 12. Byzantine Vision and Medieval Inquiry: Summary Comparison, page 261; and the glossaries, pages 346-356, with a few deletions and additions.

Excerpts adapted with actual dialogue correct quotes from UNCOMMON THERAPY: The Psychiatric Techniques Of Milton H. Erickson, M.D., by Jay Haley, by permission of Jay Haley and W.W. Norton & Company, Inc., copyright (c) 1986, 1973, by Jay Haley.

The diagram of Park City Center, Lancaster, Pennsylvania, is reproduced from a glossy by White Oak Printing Co. and used with the kind permission of Harry Grandon and the Park City Center.

The figure of the method used in presenting two cognitive tasks simultaneously, one to each hemisphere is from THE INTEGRATED MIND (New York: Plenum Press, 1978), by Michael S. Gazzaniga and Joseph E. LeDoux, Figure 42 on page 149, and used with permission of Plenum Publishers and Michael S. Gazzaniga, Ph.D.

The figure of the primate forebrain is from Paul D. MacLean, "The Brain in Relation to Empathy and Medical Education," *Journal of Nervous and Mental Disease* 144 (1967):374-382 and is used by kind permission of Paul D. MacLean, M.D., and (c) by Williams & Wilkins.

The illustrations by Keith McBarron were adapted from the following:

The brain from STRUCTURE OF THE HUMAN BRAIN: A Photographic Atlas by Stephen J. DeArmond, Medeline M. Fusco, and Maynard M. Dewey (New York: Oxford University Press, 1974), page 5 Lateral surface of the brain-actual size.

Thomas F. Mathews, THE BYZANTINE CHURCHES OF IS-
TANBUL: A PHOTOGRAPHIC SURVEY (University Park,
PA: The Pennsylvania State University Press, 1976): St. Sophia
general view of the east end, 1909. Photo Sir I. Benjamin Stone
Collection, The Birmingham Public Libraries, with the sides
cropped and the minarets and large tree in the center removed,
page 284:31-28; and the main portal from the outer narthex looking into the nave M6416A, with the people removed, page 288:31-
38.

Emile Mâle, CHARTRES, trans. by Sarah Wilson. Icon Edition
(New York: Harper & Row, Publishers, 1983): 109. North Portal,
Central Bay, St. John the Baptist, St. Peter, page 140, and 139.
Jean de Beauce's spire, page 181.

Evanston, Illinois

June 1988

Table of Contents

INTRODUCTION

I write to understand belief in God in light of brain research. Thus I describe what people believe about God in terms of what we are learning about the brain. I am finding that the brain makes our convictions about the universe--around us and inside us--plausible. And because of that believability we have knowledge with which to live life more fully.

Two problems focus that task for me:

differences in the beliefs people hold, and

differences in men and women.

These differences take many forms. I deal with two: architecture as a way people express what they believe, and what women and men take to be reality.

In Chapter One on "Architectural Images of The Center of Life," I present prime examples of how people have expressed their beliefs historically, at least in the Judeo-Christian tradition of The West.

The great dome of St. Sophia in Istanbul hovers over the landscape, embracing everything under its canopy as it lifts humanity up into the light of God. Here we see the Byzantine world in all its splendor--a harmonization of Christian vision and Roman government. Everything is of a piece, a whole, a mosaic of life and meaning. The locus of the Holy can be found anywhere and everywhere. The universe radiates with the glory of the Risen Christ.

In contrast, the great spires of Chartres Cathedral soar upward, calling people to the altar on which God sacrificed Himself on behalf of fallen humanity. Here we see the Medieval world in all its majesty--a reconciliation of spirit and matter. Everything is ordered, logical, explained. The locus of the Holy is known. Life is a pilgrimage to the place of redemption.

Whether the locus of what matters is dispersed as in the dome-like or fixed as in the spire-like, each attempts to center life. And always The Center has been sacred, the place in which we move from one dimension of reality to another. The shopping mall appears to be a way of expressing that Center by bringing order to our contemporary sprawl.

What might lead people to build such contrasting structures as dome, spire, and mall? What might have produced such different emphases in belief? How might we account for their similarities as well as their differences?

I propose that brain research illumines these questions. Architecture reflects belief, and people formalize belief in theology. Patterns of belief disclose different ways people process information. Instead of searching the universe around us for clues to these patterns I suggest we turn to the universe within. Our brain provides a locus for understanding these places and patterns of the Holy.

In Chapter Two on "In The Image And Likeness of God," I turn to the puzzling stress women and men experience in their lives together. No amount of rhetoric can lessen the pain of those differences nor any amount of goodwill eliminate the persistence of that strain. Women and men differ, not only their bodies, but also in how and what they believe.

Are the gender differences more illusionary than real? More secondary than primary? A matter of individual variations rather than gender itself? These are the questions I explore.

If the differences between men and women make a difference that constitutes a significant difference, how can the brain help us understand those differences? How do the differences develop? What keeps them going? More importantly, how can these differences enhance life instead of undermining it?

As with the question of belief, so with the question of gender--I propose that current research on the human brain helps address the differing realities of women and men. The genetic structure shapes our bodies as much as our beliefs. "Anatomy is destiny" has been a painful political slogan we must reject. At the same time anatomy (by which I mean the integration of genetic givens and cultural influences in each individual) makes for differences between the sexes, and those differences make for humanity as a species, and humanity as a species--male-and-female--is created in the image and likeness of God (Genesis 1:27).

I believe the brain sheds light on humanity as a species, in a universe believed to be created and ordered by God. Issues of architecture and gender are good examples of how people struggle to make sense of their world. I use these issues to illustrate how new understanding of the brain can lessen old struggles and direct us to more life together. The material reflects much that has led me to write about *The Brain and Belief*. In the rest of the book I explore what we are learning about the brain, how that makes belief understandable in empirical terms, and how brain and belief together can help us live more fully the life God has imaged in us as *homo sapiens*.

Having illustrated the problem of making sense of differences in architectural images and gender, in Chapter Three I describe results of experiments with split brain patients, those who have had the connections between their left and right hemispheres cut. Close attention to the subtle deficits which appeared in these patients provides evidence for distinguishing between the interpretive processing of the left brain and an imaginative processing in the right brain. For readers who might want to understand the empirical evidence and my speculations from a base in experience I provide a few exercises directed to heighten awareness of the two modes of consciousness.

In Chapter Four I explore the brain from the perspective of emergent evolution. The double mind turns out to be a brain of three minds. I detail the contrast between the older levels of brain organization--the instinctual reptilian brain and the emotional mammalian brain--and the newer level of brain organization, namely, the two hemispheres of the cerebral cortex. The older brain works in a nonconscious subsymbolic way, while the newer brain works consciously and symbolically. Only a rationalistic bias and an artificial distinction would argue for the new brain being "more important" than the older brain.

The old mammalian brain bridges--and integrates--genetic inheritance and human cognition. The issue is that of knowledge, what specialists call "epistemology." In Chapter Five I consider the nature and origin of what we know and how we know what we know. Traditionally that concern has been confined to philosophy. In recent years it has become the focus of the cognitive sciences as well.

The classical western view conceived of reality as substantial and independent of people, permanent and eternal, objective and the essence of things. The new view understands reality in a way which combines bodily knowing with mental representation. One researcher calls this view "experiential realism" (Lakoff 1987). The new view of mind--inclusive of subcortical as well as cortical input--replaces the old rational view of mind which restricted the brain to the neocortex, and more particularly to the rational interpretive activity of the left hemisphere.

I build on this newer view of cognition by shifting the focus of inquiry about the nature of the universe, ourselves, and God from the philosophical concern with Being to an empirical concern with Brain. Instead of thinking of God as Being Itself or the Power of Being, as natural theology did, I suggest that we think of God as the meaning-making reality of our various realities--my view of a new form of natural theology in an empirical mode. In this approach there is a dialectic between the phenomenological and the empirical, between cognition as strictly rational and cognition as subcortically based. The shift in focus enables us to move conceptually--and thereby intelligibly--back and forth between science and theology. As we understand the importance of the "old" brain, we can appreciate the scope of the "new" mind.

Chapter Six describes how the new view of mind can lead to a new understanding of belief. I contend there can be no brain without belief and no belief without brain. Even though we use different words to emphasize different aspects of brain and belief, they are one and the same. Different beliefs reflect different cognitive processes, as I analyze in the two creation narratives in Genesis-- the disrupted universe of Chapters 2-3 and the supportive universe of Genesis 1. These beliefs, in turn, reflect basic evolutionary plots related to the balance--and integration--of concern with the self and concern with others.

Admittedly, in linking brain and belief together in this way I am speculating. Yet such an association makes religious intuitions about life conceptually understandable. The assumptions and explanations we used to make reality sensible are tied in with our experience as living organisms, and in so doing our actions are judged by the way we adapt--or fail to adapt--to the requirements of evolution.

In a personal response to these speculations, my editorial consultant Barbara Stinchcombe wrote an extended account of her own growth and development as a person of belief and unbelief. Her story serves to bridge the gap between empirical evidence and my interpretive explanation. Barbara's description--really her testimony--came as an unexpected "gift" in the midst of this difficult task of making sense of the ways we believe.

Chapters Seven "Mechanisms of Belief" and Eight "Patterns of Belief" are heavy reading. They are the most abstract because in them I map--according to the landscape of the old brain/new mind- -how people in The West have conceived of reality. Some have affirmed the worth of what is--in themselves and in the world around them--believing it to be valuable as it is. Mostly they savor life. Others have sought to transform what is--in themselves and in the world around them--believing it to be deficient at best or distorted at worse. Mostly they try to save the world. Although still others have lived as though they were responsible for caring for the world, the distinction between savoring (affirming) and saving (transforming) has been viewed as a dichotomy, an either savor or save, not savor-and-save. In detailing the mindscape of belief I describe ways knowledge of the brain can make the task of living easier.

In "Our Sensory Systems As Language" (Chapter Nine) and "Toward A New Creativity of Being" (Chapter Ten), I develop those insights more specifically and more systematically. Then, for the curious reader I offer suggestions for further study.

Making Meaning

In addition to giving a preview of my ideas, I want also to convey somewhat impressionistically what the book is about. We are story telling creatures. Our stories are ways we make sense of life. Our universe, thereby, is not simply an impersonal environment. Rather, with stories we make it very much a personal world of meaning and the making of meaning. Because of our stories, nothing is simply what it is in itself; everything is ever and always part of something more than itself. I believe it is that "something more" which characterizes who each of us is individually and who humanity is collectively.

So I tell two stories to suggest my own belief about reality. They are about a folk prophet named Nasrudin, who reputedly lived in Persia in the thirteenth century.

Every week Nasrudin loaded up his donkey with merchandise and trudged to the frontier to cross over into Greece. The border patrol would stop him and demand, "What are you doing?"

"I'm smuggling."

With that the customs official would search his gear in an effort to find the smuggled goods--to no avail. He would have to let him go.

The next week Nasrudin would load up his donkey again, arrive at the border, and be accosted by the official: "What are you doing?"

"I'm smuggling."

And every time the official would search his gear--to no avail. Again Nasrudin would go his way. And again he would trudge home after disposing of the goods.

This went on week after week, month after month, for years. Eventually, the official retired and moved to Cairo. There on the street he bumped into Nasrudin who, by this time, had become a wealthy merchant. The ex-official could restrain his frustration no longer.

"You have bugged me all these years," he snarled. "Now that we are away from the long arm of the law, what was it you were smuggling?"

"Quite simple. Donkeys" (Shah [1964, 1969] 1971, 59).

I will refer to this story occasionally because it reminds us of the subtlety of the obvious, the obvious being that which is there but not seen by us. Not unlike the customs official who exhausted himself in his search for contraband, never finding the smuggled merchandise among the bundles on the donkey's back because those bundles were the camouflage for the real article itself, we search for God only to discover that what we were searching for was in front of us all the time.

Augustine voiced my point in religious language when he confessed, "Where, then, wast thou [O God] and how far from me? . . . I sought after thee, but not according to the understanding of the mind . . . but only after the guidance of my physical senses. Thou wast more inward to me than the most inward part of me; and higher than my highest reach" (Augustine 1955, Bk. III, VI,68).

The subtlety of the obvious is the reality of God's presence. God is in our midst, in our minds, in our brains, in our world. Or, perhaps more accurately, "made in the image and likeness of God," we are to reproduce our kind (Genesis 1:27b-28) and be responsible for ("have dominion over") the universe in which we find ourselves (Genesis 1:26).

The reality of our situation--the brain--is immediately in front of us. In other words, the brain is the tool with which we believe. The universe within us is the clue to the universe around us. We need not look elsewhere--outside of ourselves--we need only turn to that which carries the goods of our world, the source of our imaginings, the origin of our beginning and the destiny of our becoming. Donkeys or brains or beliefs or God, my point is the same: what we are looking for is right before our eyes, if only we have eyes to see and a mind to believe.

The second story is like the first. One night Nasrudin found himself in a tea house, caught between two men arguing over a basic fact of the universe. One claimed, "The sun is more important than the moon." The other countered, "The moon is more important than the sun."

Neither was making headway against the other. Finally they turned to Nasrudin. "Which is more important?" they beseeched him. "The sun or the moon?"

"It's quite simple," he announced. "The moon is more important than the sun."

With that the "moon" man stopped thinking. But the "sun" man continued the argument. "How can you say 'the moon is more important than the sun'?" he demanded.

"It's quite simple, as I said." Nasrudin replied. "The moon is more important than the sun . . . because . . . at night we need the light more" (Shah [1964,1969] 1971, 76).

Perhaps you smile at his rationale. If so, why? What tickled your fancy? Most people report something about the "cleverness" of his answer, the "absurdity" of his answer, the "complementarity" of the sun and the moon. As with smuggling, the argument reveals the foolishness of so many of the contrasts we make-up about life. There is no way we can separate sun and moon, day and night, noontime and twilight. These are distinguishable, yes; but, they are not divisible. They belong to each other; they are part of a greater whole; they are ever and always variations within a single reality.

This story of the moon and the sun suggests the integrity of complexity. Whether we divide the world into good and bad, female and male, the West and the East, religious and nonreligious, spirit and matter, body and soul--or any other dualism, dichotomy, and polarity--we are arguing about a product of our human imagining. Reality itself is whole, an integrity (Sanders 1987b). No matter how suggestive our imaginings may be, they are variations on the simple fact of a functioning system, one which is unified and unifying, emerging and evolving, ever-present and ever-surprising. We are part of a universe in which everything fits together.

Through the centuries the ideas of the physical and the purposeful, of the sensory and the spiritual, of body and mind have been elevated to permanent entities, each substantial in itself and each independent of the other. The complexity may be simpler than we have realized. The subtlety may be more obvious than we have discerned.

In investigating the relationship of brain and belief, I am suggesting that the complexity of the opposition between physical matter and psychic meaning has more wholeness than people have understood. I am proposing that the relatedness is more accessible than we have suspected. In what follows, remember the impact of Nasrudin's stories about "donkeys" and "the moon is more important than the sun."

We tell stories as a way of making meaning. These folk tales illustrate how we fool each other and how we try to make sense of the universe. In *Romans*, St. Paul tells a story of the struggle many of us experience between the desire to act one way and the drive which causes us to act in an opposite way:

> I cannot understand my own behaviour. *I fail to carry out the things I want to do, and I find myself doing the very things I hate* . . . though the will to do what is good is in me, the performance is not, with the result that instead of doing the good things I want to do, I carry out the sinful things I do not want. When I act against my will, then it is not my true self doing it, but sin which lives in me.
>
> In fact, this seems to be the rule, that every single time I want to do good it is something evil that comes to hand. *In my inmost self I dearly love God's Law, but I can see that my body follows a different law that battles against the law which my reason dictates. . .*
>
> What a wretched man I am! Who will rescue me from this body doomed to death? Thanks be to God through Jesus Christ our Lord!
>
> In short, it is I who with my reason serve the Law of God, and no less I who serve in my unspiritual self the law of sin.
>
> (Romans 7:15-25 JB [emphasis added])

Whether Paul is telling about his own struggle or simply voicing that of others is debatable. However, most of us have experienced--and do experience--that pain and that pull. One side of us feels one way; another side of us fights for the opposite.

As with architectural images and gender differences, the brain makes such struggle understandable in both experiential and empirical ways. The double mind provides a way to conceive of what the struggle is about, to describe the confusion, and most of all to reduce the strain. The task, of course, is not new. People have always tried to make sense of such divisions within themselves. In that respect, our age is no different.

What is different is that we are demystifying reality. In the past, conflicting forces were experienced as competing gods and goddesses, humanity against divinity, me against the demonic, the divine against the "old me." Today we approach such struggles as internal processes, not alien power. Yet even to put the issue that way obscures the richness of myth and metaphor on the one hand and science and explanation on the other.

Different Languages

Some people deal with that longing for wholeness with philosophical and theological language. For instance, they speak of the meaning of human nature and human destiny. Others deal with that longing by means of physical and positivistic approaches, such as identifying physical forces, biochemical processes, and biosocial interactions. While we approach issues differently, the questions remain similar.

How can we be the human beings that we are? How can we be part of the human family to which we belong? What are our resources and what makes for renewal? Is the context in which we live "gracious" or "abusive?" Are we simply thrown into an empty void or are we part of an emerging sensibility?

Traditionally, religious people have turned to a cosmic connection to make sense of confusion in themselves and their world. God, however that reality has been understood, has been part and parcel of life on this planet. Alternatively, nonreligious people have looked to themselves and their ability to identify and control the forces of nature in overcoming confusion in themselves and their world. Order and chaos, however that balance has been understood, has been the focus of their efforts in the service of life.

In our time, new knowledge is generating new possibilities--possibilities that avoid a sharp division between a divine mystery and a human mastery. Patterns of belief are more explainable in light of brain processes, at least so it seems to me and others. In different ways, empirical explanation and religious conviction are clarifying the gracious givens of human life and the genuine choices in human becoming. Our many minds are beginning to make sense of our many meanings. And that sensibility offers promise of our living more intentionally and more intelligibly. Such intelligibility, I contend, arises from our being part of a vaster universe than we can ever fully know or command.

I combine what we are learning about the brain with what we have known in belief. Whether we start with the brain or belief we are dealing with ourselves--ourselves as physical reality and ourselves as purposive reality. I believe that our physical reality--that is, our brain--**is** purposive reality, and that our purposive reality--that is, belief--**is** physical reality. The physical and the purposive in our brain are not two realities; they are **one** reality. To separate them violates the very nature of reality itself.

I realize that such conviction is at odds with both a view of the universe as only physical and a view of the universe as really spiritual. Classically, body and soul, brain and mind, humanity and divinity, matter and meaning, the physical and the conceptual, the sensory and the spiritual, or whatever contrasts people have used to talk about themselves and the universe have been taken to be objective, independent of humanity itself. Today, new knowledge of ourselves helps us understand that the words we use to describe our experience are mental representations of experience and not entities in themselves. Whether couched in the language of theology or science, the ways we talk about ourselves, the universe, and God are a blend of bodily experience, leaps of imagination, and conscious reason (Johnson 1987).

We are object-seeking creatures and meaning-making animals. We feel, imagine, conceive, and give voice to the sense that we make of our senses. To that end we draw upon both the experiences which constrain us and the imaginings by which we create meaning. We are part of what is, even as we construct the reality of "what is."

CHAPTER ONE

ARCHITECTURAL IMAGES OF THE CENTER OF LIFE:

ST. SOPHIA AND CHARTRES

Adam/Eve, where are you?
(Genesis 3:9)

Oh that I knew where I might find God?
(Job 23:3 KJ)

Not on this mountain
nor in Jerusalem
(John 4:19-23)

Recently, a suburban pastor complained to me about a gigantic shopping mall being built near him. Then he observed, "People come together but they do not gather" (Nelson 1987).

What is the significance -- the human and therefore psychic or spiritual significance -- of the shopping mall? Teen-agers congregate; retirees wander; shoppers search; friends agree to "meetcha at the mall." Is it simply what that pastor lamented: coming together without gathering? Or is the phenomenon something more?

The shopping mall is bringing order to the suburban sprawl. Like cosmic magnets they are drawing more people, more of the time, than any other "space" in the North American scene. Studies show that people spend the largest amount of time, outside their home and job, in malls. To the discerning eye of Religious Studies

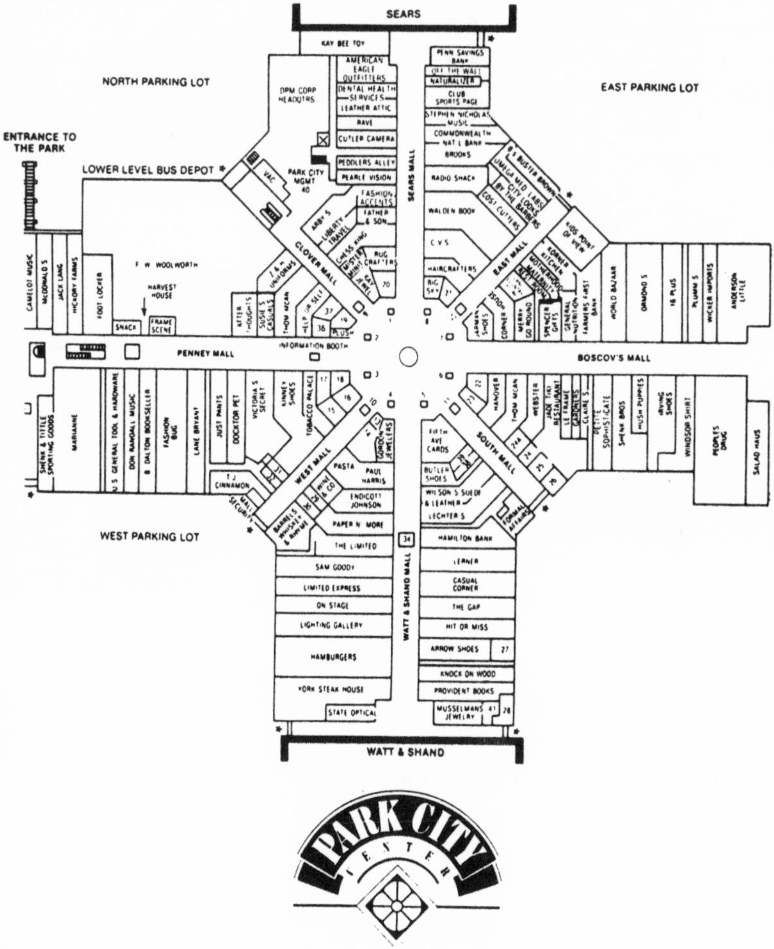

FIGURE 1. Park City Center, Lancaster, PA.

Professor Ira G. Zepp, Jr. the shopping mall has become the Ceremonial Center of Urban America (1986).

The shopping complex appears to be satisfying our archetypal longing for centeredness and festivity, for community and carnival. The Mall has taken on the qualities of sacred space, the qualities of the Center of meaning which organizes life together -- circles and crosses, squares and pathways, fountains and trees, flags and monuments (see Figure 1). The architectural space is quadrilateral. Like the typical basilica or cathedral, the mall is shaped in the fourfold form of a mandala, which is a symbol for wholeness, completeness, fulfillment. There are the many circles of rose-like cathedral windows, and all paths lead to the center.

Not only does The Mall constitute sacred space, it also offers sacred time. It presents festival time -- play and performance, eating and relaxing, sanctuary from the hustle and bustle of everyday obligation. There are seasonal celebrations -- special sales to use commercial language. There are evidences of nature -- ever flowing water, ever blooming plants, ever splendid light -- special effects to attract the wayfarer.

As Zepp concludes: the shopping mall expresses in concrete form the three impulses of religion -- the need to represent life symbolically, the need to ritualize major events, and the "desire to be in a community. . . . Quadrilateral architecture, calendrical rituals, replications of natural settings, and attempts to be people places and objects of pilgrimage, all illustrate homo religosus" (Zepp 1986, 150).

> I'm not certain whether the developer or architect or customer or clerk is altogether conscious of it, but the centeredness of the mall is a way most of us find a certain microcosmic reflection of the world. The theory is that a square or circle or cross is a way of saying life is fundamentally safe. It's a miniaturization of the universe (Zepp quoted by Cole 1986, 12).

Our world is high-speed, fast-service, endless choices. As a consumer-driven society, we have plenty of places for people to come together -- anonymously, individually, isolated from each other. We have less and less space for intimate gathering for personal sharing, simply for breathing. Space for our common good is bureaucratized -- public buildings with busy corridors during the day and deserted hallways during the night. Space for common caring is segregated into shelters for the homeless -- church basements and cinderblock fortresses. Open spaces let us escape from each other; secluded spaces protect us from having to be with others, especially others who are different from us -- the marginal and the outcast.

In these patterns of impersonal space, of bureaucratized space, of segregated space, of protected space, of inaccessible space, even of shopping mall space, no space remains sacred. All space stands exposed to the erosion of meaning and the invasion of privacy. Yet we are made for meaning. We long for relatedness. We want to go where life matters.

How we organize space reveals what matters to us (Giedion 1964; 1967; Prak 1968; Zevi 1957). More specifically, architecture can be understood as outward and visible images of our inward and spiritual mindsets (Eliade [1954] 1959, 6-11). What we tear down and what we erect -- what we close off and what we open up -- all reveal patterns of human community. Even within the most functional building, latent powers of relatedness and meaning exert their influence. The truth is: *we build what we are, and we are what we build.* By our buildings we transform an impersonal environment into a world full of meaning.

When Humanoids Stood Up

The beginnings of "human" activity have been identified with our standing upright (Kolb and Whishaw [1980] 1985, 80-97). Humanoids stopped scurrying around on all fours, grunting and growling, sniffing and smelling. Instead, our ancestors stood up. They began to use their front paws as instruments with which to take hold of objects. Instead of gutteral sounds with coded messages, throats and vocal cords developed specialized sounds. Those sounds became the foundation of the most earthy and the most abstract expressions of subtle and sophisticated information (Goodenough 1987). As the primary source of information, our eyes became more important than our nose. Instead of simply smelling the environment, we surveyed a world (Tillich 1987, 199-203).

Once on our feet the vertical perspective replaced the horizontal perspective (Giedion 1964, 435-439). The upright stance organized what mattered. No longer were all directions of equal importance. No longer were the rest and repose -- equilibrium if you will -- of the horizontal as compelling as the remote and the challenging, Once on our feet, we moved around. No longer were we restricted to a narrow territory marked out by our reptilian brain. We turned our eyes outward, upward, forward. We longed to venture beyond the horizon, into the clouds, beyond the sun and the moon and the stars. The physical environment became the vehicle of our quest for meaning.

From the Egyptian obelisks to the megolithic Stonehenge circles, the upright pointed us from earth to heaven. In the presence of the vertical, our attention moved "from earthly existence to the abode of the gods" (Giedion 1964, 440). Our human presence initiated our quest for divine reality.

Monumental architecture shaped that symbolic quest (Giedion 1964, 350). In the Babylonian mindset, the ziggurats -- those temple towers in the form of a terraced pyramid of successively higher receding storied steps -- were stairways to the gods. Those massive structures stood within the city of the living. They made the summit of our search accessible to all. In contrast, to the Egyptian mindset the pyramids served as obstacles to the gods. Those massive structures rose in desert places, apart from lived life. They made the doorway to the gods inaccessible to all.

Whether part of the ongoing or apart from the everyday, monumental structures focused the community's psychic energy and physical economy. People used the vertical, upright perspective to translate their vision of the meaning of life into visible form.

Space, thereby, discloses the way we orient ourselves to what we regard as really real. The shape of space and the use of space tell us who we are and what we are about (Tillich 1987, 82-84). As such, space symbolizes our mindset and makes concrete our values. It reveals both our conscious and our nonconscious views of the world. We impose our worldviews -- our "human" worlds -- upon the physical environment. As we interpret the ways we structure space, so we identify our views of what matters most in our experience.

To say what space says, however, we must make the implicit pattern of lines and shapes, of outside and inside, of distance and closeness, of definiteness and openness explicit. We have to ask specifically: what is this particular space saying to us about what matters to us? In working with dreams, we have to say in words what we see with our mind's eye. The same applies to architecture. We have to translate what we experience in our bodies and see with our eyes into ideas in our heads and words in our mouths.

All buildings, and their spaces, reflect aspects of our views of life. Some buildings, however, convey more of that meaning than others. I regard such special buildings as archetypal. That is, they carry the powerful nonconscious meanings which express our basic values. We put into visual form the *human* reality by which we live.

I suggest two architectural forms which are archetypal -- or prototypical -- of our quest to connect physical space with its spiritual significance (Ashbrook 1984c, 109-123). One is the dome of the basilica of Hagia Sophia in Istanbul (Ashbrook, 1984c, 124-

177); the other is the spire of the cathedral at Chartres in France (Ashbrook 1984c, 178-258).

The dome and the spire, I contend, reflect the two basic strategies by which the brain deals with the world: namely, the all-at-once imaginative responsesiveness of the right hemisphere and the step-by-step analytic rationality of the left hemisphere. These physical images express our spiritual perceptions. They re-present how we perceived reality and how we organize reality. They orient us to the locus of the holy -- The Center -- "the zone of absolute reality" (Eliade [1954] 1959, 12-21).

In religious language, the dome and the spire are the dwelling places of the Most High God. As such, the buildings reveal the Holy of Holies, the ultimacy of our ultimate concern. Beyond their historical significance, each offers a glimpse of more univer-sal meaning. That is why I suggest they are archetypal. In them we learn about what matters most in human experience.

I describe the archetypal meaning of the dome and the spire by combining patterns of belief, brain processes, and cultural values. These two configurations of different cultures paralleled each other for a thousand years. Despite variations through the cen-turies, and despite variations across cultures, they crystallized in stone two distinct ways of connecting heaven and earth: the expan-siveness of a domelike mindset and the intensiveness of a spirelike mindset. After contemplating these two patterns we can return to the various spaces of our lives with new understanding and renewed intention.

The Dome: Byzantine Vision[1]

From the outside, Hagia Sophia's rough exterior belies its ex-quisite interior. The great dome hovers over the landscape reminding us twentieth century folk of a vehicle from outer space (Figure 2). Nor are we alone in our association of the dome and the heavens.

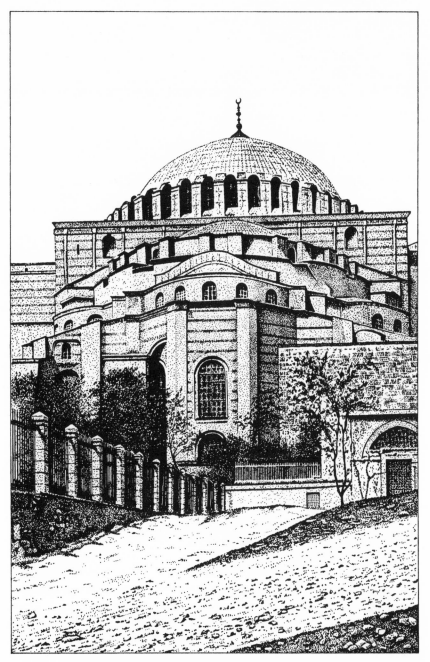

FIGURE 2. East end of St. Sophia.

When the building was completed in 562 C.E., Paul the Silentiary celebrated the event with a poem: "There overhead," he wrote, "looming vast in the shadowy air, arches the rounded helm of the heavenly house/Like unto the burnished roof of heaven" (quoted by Kahler 1967, 11). Nor was Paul alone. In a similar poetic mode, Procopius, the Greek historian of Late Antiquity, described the building as

> . . . a spectacle of marvelous beauty, overwhelming to those who see it . . . soaring to a height to match the sky, and, as if surging up from amongst the other buildings it stands on high and looks down upon the remainder of the city . . . dominating it . . . exulting in an indescribable beauty . . . it seems somehow to float in the air on no firm basis . . . Yet actually it is braced with exceptional firmness . . . (Procopius [1940] 1961, I:i,21,34; VII:13, 17-19).

Despite the massiveness of the structure, only the dome draws our attention. The building appears to expand-and-embrace at one and the same time. It stands there bold-and-simple, subtle yet sure, majestic while austere, massive-though-mysterious. That splendor of dome and half-domes, rising up as waves to the sky, rests upon an intuited base of belief that included the whole of the created realm. Everything nestled under its wings. It reached out to embrace everyone and everything.

People could enter the building from any side. No one entrance stood out as "the only way." The many entrances conveyed openness in the society and the open quality of human nature. All who belonged were capable of taking part in every part of its life.

From the western side of the structure two sets of five doors opened onto three sets of three doors. An outer narthex and an inner narthex stretched the entire length of the building. The fact that the inner narthex is twice as deep and twice as high as the outer one only heightens our sense of something marvelous un-

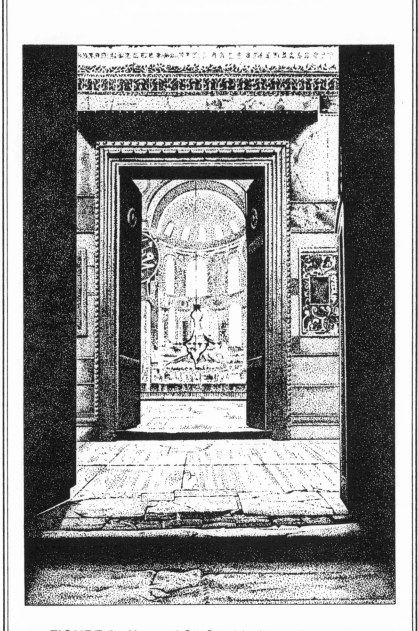

FIGURE 3. Nave of St. Sophia from the narthex.

folding before us. The cross-vaulting and ceiling pull us forward, carrying us on waves of mounting expectation. The combination of many entrances, opening into successive narthexes, and the final glimpsing of ourselves in the midst of exalted and expansive spaciousness creates a sense of our being borne by the quickening rhythm of waves cresting onto a shoreline (Figure 3).

Inside the building, space also seems to expand and embrace at one and the same time. We experience a dynamic vitality emanating from its open vastness. Again I turn to Procopius to convey the awesomeness of that vision of the really Real. He spoke of the building's infinite detail, an intricacy inviting infinite wonder in the soul of the observer.

> All the details, fitted together with incredible skill in mid-air and floating off from each other and resting only on the parts next to them, produce a single and most extraordinary harmony . . . and yet [they] do not permit the spectator to linger much over the study of any one of them, but each detail attracts the eye and draws it on irresistibly to itself (Procopius [1940] 1962, VII:21).

One quality looms more prominently than any other in that inner space. It is wondrous light. Above the central door to that inner vastness is a mosaic of Christ. The inscription reads: "Peace be unto you. I am the light of the world." Even though the mosaic is a much later addition to the inner narthex, the message was central to the eyes of the believers. For Byzantium, light constituted the first-created element in the world. So, within the spacious cavern, light plays continuously as it filters down from above. The source of the light remains hidden, radiating, it seems, from within the space itself. Once over the threshold of the narthex and on into the open nave we are bathed in light. For the early Christians, the Light of the world shone everywhere.

This image of the one dome provided believers with a unifying vision of reality: all were included, all was affirmed, humanity was lifted up into the light of God. Thus, for the domelike mentality, words expressing light are commonplace -- illumination, enlightenment, manifestation, insight. Everything -- everywhere -- radiates with the light of the world.

Christians identified Christ as the true self. The image of Christ appears in the summit of the dome of the Middle Byzantine church even though the image is not in the dome of Hagia Sophia. The iconic image functioned to facilitate the identification of Christians with Christ. As the Risen Lord, Christ is not a "remote cosmic ruler . . . [but] so close to the viewer that he is inside [one] for it is the true self, whole and complete, which the Christian is always becoming" (Mathews 1984, 14-16).

That Byzantine vision of Christ as the Light of the World was simple and straightforward: one citizenry obeyed one law by believing in one creed. For them, everything emanated from the triumphant Christ, the Ruler of the Universe (Mathews 1984, 16-21). And the one dome expressed that fully perfect reality.

In 335, Eusebius (ca. 263-340), bishop of Caesarea, described the Byzantine world in this way: "And thus, by the express appointment of the same God, two roots of blessing, the Roman empire, and the doctrine of Christian piety, sprang up together for the benefit of [humanity]" (quoted by Magoulias 1970, 1). Politics and piety fused as a political machine and a religious explanation combined. Because the patriarch anointed the emperor, the coronation expressed the will of God. The earthly realm and the heavenly realm mirrored each other. To the eye of believers, the Christian Universe and the Greco-Roman world were one.

People could enter into that structure which embodied God's Holy Wisdom as it was understood by those early believers, therefore, through many entrances. Many ways suggested their belief in the open quality of human nature and the open structures in society.

Life was an everflowing process, an ascending to God and a communing with God. Everyone was encouraged to enter into, to be part of, to be lifted up into that transfigured reality which had transformed darkness into marvelous light.

Because everything belonged together, under the one dome, the locus of the holy was, as the Late Antiquity scholar Peter Brown put it, "tantalizingly always ambiguous" (Brown 1976, 11-16). God could be present as fully in a physician in Alexandria as in a St. Anthony in the desert or in a farmer in a rural village. Epiphanies -- God appearances -- came suddenly, unexpectedly, repeatedly. Whether in the natural order, the communal order, or the cosmic order, the really Real disclosed itself in surprising and varied ways. In the reality of the domelike, the holy escaped confinement. And we can see that ever-flowing forth as fully in the intricate ornamental lines of the pillars as we can hear it in the doctrinal statements of the theologians.

The hovering dome included all. In the building itself no structural line sharply divides the piers, the columns, or the stoa. No status sharply divided person from person or group from group. The throne stood open to all, regardless of a person's rank, fortune, or ancestry. Open space in architecture expressed open roles in society. Anyone could play a big part in the divine drama. Every person and every part converged to create one magnificent mosaic of divine meaningfulness. The wondrous light of the basilica radiated the pervasive presence of Wisdom.

Unreflective Imagination

The Byzantine mindset lived in a world of its own imagining. Circumstances of history, observations of nature, or rational inquiry seldom modified this quickened sense of transcendence. Believers plated Constantinople with gold because, for them, their city **was** the New Jerusalem. All was light and in Light there was no darkness at all.

Their right brain process, I would suggest, lacked the perspective that comes with realistic observation. They saw only what they imagined they saw -- the holiness of the Holy and nothing else. Theirs was a myopic optimism, not unlike the "polishing" we know is associated with strong right hemisphere dominance.[2] They saw life as better than it was. Few difficulties, fewer disturbances, no disruption of the Divine Presence. All was Light -- holy light, holy wisdom, wholly Christ.

This myopia accounts for their lack of a sense of sin, I believe. God did not need to restore a fallen humanity to right relationships. Right relationships already existed.

Yet violence marked every transfer of political power. I find the facts astounding:

> Of the 109 sovereigns, 65 were assassinated, 12 died in convent or prison, 3 died of hunger, 18 were castrated or had their eyes put out, their noses or hands cut off, and the rest were poisoned, suffocated, strangled, stabbed, thrown down from the top of a column or ignominiously hunted down. In 1,058 years there were 65 revolutions of palace, street or barracks and 65 dethronements . . . Byzantium . . . was an absolute monarchy tempered by assassination (Guerdan [1957] 1962, 135).

Because the mentality of the people lacked rational procedures -- the step-by-step processing of left brain activity -- no procedure guided political changes. Every transition in imperial authority meant disruption of everything, everywhere. People started over everytime, from the beginning, with a new beginning that was not a beginning, for all was fulfilled in the hovering embrace of the dome.

Even when Constantinople fell to the Turks in 1453, the political reality of Byzantium became the universal state of Orthodoxy. A spiritual empire replaced the physical empire. "True" reality continued in the Orthodox Church of Eastern Christianity even though its earthen vessel of the Byzantine Empire was no more. The domelike mindset polished everything with optimism, a quality I have associated with its gold-plating obsession. That bias kept the Byzantine imagination from perceiving anything other than its own imaginings.

I conclude from this pattern that Byzantium lacked the vigilant observation of left brain activity.

Domelike Expansiveness

Having noted this deficiency -- and its consequence -- I want to emphasize the fact that the dome hovered brilliantly over a portion of western civilization for a thousand years. Furthermore, that domelike quality of God manifesting God unpredictably still quickens the imaginative eye of faith. It reminds us of the expansive openness of the relational process, arising in and through the activity of our right hemisphere and the relaxing response of the autonomic nervous system.

The domelike mentality inspires us by its exquisite leaps of imagination. It is exactly these leaps that create believers. Faith is such a leap, even when one knows one does not know. The leap renews our *human* spirit. Without it we remain earthbound and culturebound -- ethnocentric -- stunted caricatures of who we are. No longer Godlike.

The relational strategy of the archetypal dome makes for diversity and expansiveness. It affirms everything that is, which means belief in an indicative mode. What "is" is the "really real." In the here-and-now we know the living God -- God in all, God through all, God with all. That relational reality connects us with the whole created world through the functioning of our limbic system. We care about each other and we care about ourselves because we experience ourselves to be part and parcel of a caring cosmic context.

St. Symeon, the New Theologian, made the point I am trying to make. Mystical experience provides the source for rational explanation. Said Symeon: "Within all of human nature [God] placed a loving power so that the rational nature of [humanity] might be helped by the natural power of love" (quoted by Magoulias 1970, 78).

I find an even more majestic expression of this archetypal mindset in Nicolas Cabasilas (14th century), the last of the great Byzantine mystics. He avoided an otherworldy asceticism by making piety solely an issue of inner intention. I understand that inner intention to mean activating the whole brain and not simply allowing the right brain, or the left for that matter, to dominate. Cabasilas wrote:

> The law of the Spirit, which is love of God, is a law of friendship and gratitude. To follow this law one need not expend effort or expense or shed perspiration . . . Nor is it necessary to leave your work or go to out-of-the-way places . . . Because there is no place where God is absent, it is not possible for God not to be with us . . . [God] will come to us even if we are evil, because God is good (quoted by Magoulias 1970, 84).

The domelike mentality -- right brain activity if you will allow such an inferential leap or analogy -- invites us to discover our connectedness with everyone and everything. Worldly wisdom emerges from a wondrous context. So, too, the wondrous context is fulfilled through worldly wisdom.

In the prosaic language of the neurosciences, the subsymbolic paradigm (Rumelhart et al [1986] 1987), which processes information *below* the conscious level, informs the symbolic paradigm. In turn, the symbolic paradigm, which operates *at* the level of consciousness, interprets the subsymbolic paradigm. In effect, first the intuitive, then the interpretive; first the mystical, then the worldly.

Byzantine culture presents us with a prototypical image of the meaning of life. It is the image of the dome and, by inference, all that is domelike. In the domelike we can experience an inspired confidence that links us with spiritual inclusiveness. The domelike quickens and expands reality. Truly "the earth is full of the steadfast love of the Lord" (Psalm 33:5 RSV).

The Spire: Medieval Inquiry[3]

In contrast to the inclusive embrace of the domelike, precision came to focus in Western Christianity. For the Latin believer, the locus of the holy was known (Brown 1971). God had come down and met humanity in Christ's sacrifice on the altar. In "the Gothic image" (Mâle [1913, 1958] 1972; von Simson [1956] 1974) of the medieval cathedral people believed that the invisible was made visible. Nowhere was that presence more present than in the cathedral at Chartres.

The building itself integrated Christian doctrine, formal logic, and rational inquiry. I find in its spirelike mentality archetypal intensity (Figure 4). Seen from a distance, the cathedral's spires and transepts seem, in the words of art historian Emile Mâle, "like a mighty ship about to sail on a long voyage" (Mâle [1913, 1958] 1972, 396). To the medieval person, the structure itself symbolized the ark of the world. It offered refuge from the flooding ravages of sin, of ignorance, of death. With the precise order of hierarchical authority, the spirelike mind organized the chaos of finitude.

Despite their similarity, the two towers differ (Ashbrook 1984c, 185-186). The magnificent northern spire (Figure 5) stretches 27 feet higher than the simpler southern spire. Though similar in form and function, they differed in status. The medieval rationale for organizing reality set the priority of authority: the spiritual stretched higher than the temporal. Authority "descended" from God, to pope, to priest, to laity (Ullmann 1966, 47). Two towers meant two powers -- Church and Empire. Even though the Empire insisted that papal power and imperial power paralleled each

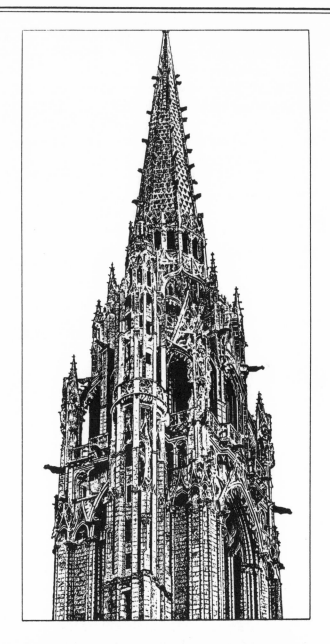

FIGURE 4. Spire, Chartres Cathedral

other, the Papacy placed itself on top. It assumed a closer connection to God. It insisted upon obedience from the Empire.

Pope Gregory the Great (590-604) laid the foundation of that mindset. Just as the universe was ordered hierarchically, so Christendom was organized hierarchically. Each power had its proper place in The Divine Scheme. Gregory made the principle clear: "Universal society could subsist by no other principle than that of a great system of order preserving its diversity of operations" (quoted by Russell 1968, 40). When Charlemagne knelt before Pope Leo III to be crowned Emperor of the Holy Roman Empire in 800, the issue was settled -- at least in the minds of the clergy. True authority consisted of two powers, in descending order, thereby establishing, in the phrase of historian R.W. Southern, "an imperial papacy" (Southern [1970] 1979, 24).

Augustine, in his book *On The Trinity*, contemplated the mystery of the redeeming work of God (Augustine [1963] 1981, esp. Bk. IV, chps. 3,4,6). What was the relationship, he asked, between Christ's one death and humanity's double death: that is, death of the body and death of the soul as a result of sin? It dawned on him that the experience of musical harmony described that reconciliation. When he heard the consonance of the octave -- that is, the musical ratio of 1:2 -- his ears heard the mystery of redemption. Musical harmony, he wrote, echoed theological truth. And that harmony found its visual transformation and equivalent in the mathematical proportion of Gothic architecture.

Like the belief structure itself, Chartres presented the trinitarian formula. Everything expressed the motif of three-in-one: two towers, one (main) entrance; two aisles, one nave; nave, chancel, apse; pier arch, triforium, clerestory; triple windows -- endless variations of that harmonization. Three articles of faith proved the existence of God. So, people could enter through three facades; each facade presented three entrances; each entrance revealed three rising bands of figures surrounding a central tympanum of recessed space. Trinitarian reality fixed every form with precision. God would be found at the altar, and only at the altar.

The building exhibits clear order: one rationale, two powers, and harmony -- despite contrasts. The towers soar into the sky, a balanced sense of aspiration as the straight lines carry one's eyes heavenward -- the spire like two limbs stretched upward in supplication. If the rib vaulting marks the first system in the Gothic system, the flying buttress marks the second (Bony 1983, 195ff). The buttresses hold together the upward thrust of the vaulting and the counterthrust to the altar -- upward yet ever forward.

In approaching the cathedral we can be bewildered by 2000 figures crowding the nine entrances (see Katzenellenbogen [1959] 1964). For the people of that earlier period no such confusion existed. Mâle described the experience of the believers:

> As one draws near [the building] one first meets the figure of Christ, as everyone born into the world meets Him on his or her voyage through life. He is the key to the riddle of life . . . The Christian is told how the world began and how it will end . . . Before one's eyes are all the people whose history it is of importance humanity should know . . . Thus the world with its history becomes intelligible.

> Side by side with the story of this vast universe, humanity's own history is written. It learns that life must be a conflict, a struggle with nature in every month of the year, a struggle with itself at every moment . . . And to those who have fought a good fight the angels in the heavens above hold out crowns . . . (Mâle [1913, 1958] 1972, 396-397).

The entrances made the message clear. Structurally, they harmonize diametrically opposed principles of design: the straight lines contain the round line; the vertical lines hold the horizontal lines; the narrow doors accentuate the larger doors; and the horizontal bands of figures link each of the three portals. Pillar figures, such as St. Peter holding the keys of the kingdom (Figure 5), signified "the pillars of humanity" (Mâle [1913, 1958] 1972, 152) even as they served as the pillars of the entrances themselves. The verticality of the pillar sculpture reinforces the stretching verticality of the spire.

Inside the building, we are dazzled by its majesty. The 130 feet of receding nave pull our eyes away from the 122 feet of soaring vault. Unlike the impressionistic mosaic of Hagia Sophia, the towers and buttresses articulate an intentional path to follow. Every part of the building contributes to a crescendo of exalted space with clear direction. We are drawn toward the altar with a sense of inevitability.

Here there are no surprises. Once we have seen the towers we know the plan. The inside re-presents the outside. Because the nave is more than twice as high as it is wide, and because it is taut by virtue of being twice the size of the aisles, we are led forward irresistibly. That intensified atmosphere defined the one "right" way to the place of The Holy.

Architecturally, then, the complex system of opposing forces represented the ambiguity of human finitude: time versus eternity, matter versus spirit, expanding curiosity versus centered faith: two towers, two powers -- One eternal, spiritual, true; the other temporal, earthly, limited. For the believers, the world was set, its forces definite, the way known. The structure made visible the invisible mind of God. The locus of the holy could be fixed, and it was fixed, by the Church, at the altar.

What had originated in the Augustinian experience of finitude culminated in the scholastic explanation of the world. The path of perception moved through a central aphorism of Anselm (1033-1109) -- "I do not seek to understand in order to believe, but I believe in order to understand" (Fairweather 1970, Anselm, Proslogion, I) -- to the reverse emphasis of Abelard (1079-1142) --

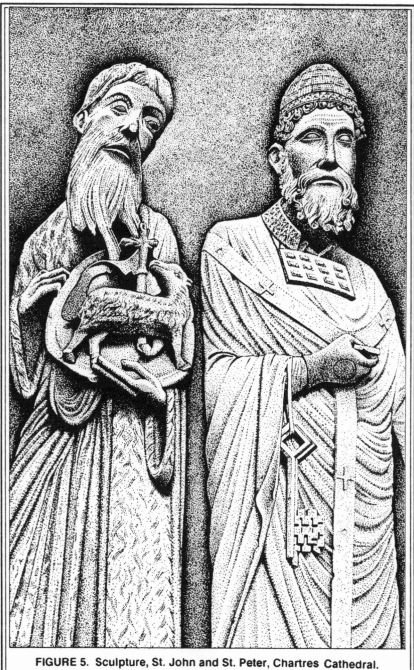

FIGURE 5. Sculpture, St. John and St. Peter, Chartres Cathedral.

"Nothing is believed unless it first be understood" (Abailard 1954, 39). The methodical method of dialectics had rigidified into Anselm's methodical faith and Abelard's methodical doubt[4] -- spatially in architecture and symbolically in belief.

In the thrust and the counterthrust of the building we can see the stance of "Yes, I believe in order to understand" and the counterstance of "No, I understand in order to believe." The rational dialectic of asymmetrical forces determined the direction and the destination of the faith journey. The design resolved the opposition of spirit and matter: theologically in doctrine, politically in papal supremacy, architecturally in the Gothic cathedral. Or, at least so it seemed to the eye of faith.

Exaggerated Rationality

Few questioned whether the rational method corresponded to physical reality. The method **was** the reality: three-in-one concentrated and controlled space. The dominating explanation of the scholastics objectified the dialectics of experience. By the thirteenth century, the breadth of interest and freshness of inquiry, which marked the humanism of the eleventh and twelfth centures, had receded. In their stead came "a gradual restriction of scope and inquiry, the first seeds of oversophisticaion . . . very largely due to the dominance of dialectic, which had almost swallowed up the other liberal arts" (Leff 1958, 168). The spirelike mentality now specified what was "urgently right."

That precision found its face in Christ as The Terrible Judge. In the tympanum at the main entrance of the cathedral he could be seen confronting humanity with its finitude and sin (Bentmann and Lickes [1970, 1978] 1979, 133). Like the person who suffers from left hemisphere damage, the medieval mind "tarnished" everything. It made life more miserable than it was, more negative than seemed necessary.[5] People lived in a state of agitated expectancy as hell loomed on every side. An oppressive pessimism permeated every nook and cranny of medieval culture.

The very method of dialectical inquiry suggests such a disturbed psychic processing, at least to me. Let me explain. The pattern of thesis/antithesis/synthesis generated competing forces. These forces clashed throughout the culture: the rival powers of pope and emperor, competing orders such as the simple Franciscans and the sophisticated Dominicans: competing pieties such as natural realism and Gothic symbolism; competing inquiries such as the empiricism of nominalism and the idealism of realism. This rigidified dialectic between what is spirit and what is matter found symbolic expression in the collapse of the Gothic cathedral itself -- literally, at both Beauvais (Bony 1961, 302) and St. Andrew's at Wells (Kessel 1964, 182). By increasing the actual height of the buildings, the balance was destroyed. In reaching higher, the buildings collapsed. Just as the cathedral structures were collapsing, so, too, was the medieval synthesis (Leff 1958, 257-303; Jonas 1974, 26; Tillich 1968, 186-209).

I infer from such evidence that the medieval mentality -- the spirelike mindset -- was disturbed. It was disturbed in terms of an hypervigilance of the left brain, triggered by the arousal of the limbic system in terms of the survival of the self. Because of that aroused vigilance, a more relaxed flow between nature and society, between individual and individual, between group and group became impossible. All that remained for a driven culture was an exaggerated rationality.

Spirelike Intentionality

Having indicated this analogy of disturbed cognition -- and its consequence -- I want to recall the fact that the spire pointed to the altar as the locus of the holy with a compelling orderliness for a thousand years. And that spirelike quality of God intentionally redeeming humanity still calls to the faithful to be faithful. The spirelike directs us to the intensity of the imperative. It instructs us on how to exercise responsibility for the whole created world (Genesis 1:28, 2:19-20).

Medieval culture suggests that the vigilant strategy of the spirelike archetype activates critical clarity. It insists upon what ought to be, which means belief in an imperative mode. What is yet to become constitutes what is "urgently right." We are exalted, though humbled. Here, then, is the prominence and necessity of a belief pattern of proclamation.

John of Salisbury made the point that the logic of obedience actually reversed the rational order of medieval authority (Fairweather 1970, 247-260). Instead of power descending from above, John claimed it proceeded up from below. The earthly power of the king "is subject to the Law of Justice." And the spiritual power of the pope depended upon the effects of policies on the welfare of the people. In effect, the people judged the politics of earthly power and the policies of spiritual power.

In this recognition of the individual human being, John reflected the humanistic expression of a freely chosen obedience. The strength of the emerging Feudalism was the shift from seeing individuals as of inferior status in the descending order of government to regarding individuals as full members of the State in an ascending order of government (Ullmann 1966, 104). As law came to rest on procedures of rational evidence and accountability, it became an instrument of liberty for high and low alike.

Furthermore, what began in mystery need not end in mastery. Left brain dominance could avoid the oppressive power of the rationalistic. The mind could be mindful of itself, its context, its source. Let me develop this point more fully.

Thomas Aquinas (1225-1274) is known as the architect of the highest spire in the medieval edifice of belief. "The Thomistic Tradition," reflective of the logic of left brain process, supposedly reigned supreme. It mastered mystery with its syllogisms. However, Thomas himself discloses greater sophistication and sensitivity (Burrell 1973; 1979).[6] He pressed intensified rationality to its limits *and* showed it wanting! This point needs more discussion.

Thomas identified the fact that we name everything only "according to our knowledge of it" (Aquinas 1945, I, 112). Then he went on to show that in a variety of ways the names we attribute to God -- good, just, love -- "fail to express [God's] mode of being because our intellect does not know [God] in this life as [God] is" (Aquinas 1945, I, 113). To state the issue crisply: the whole of Aquinas' efforts went into demonstrating what God is *not*, rather than pointing to what God is.

> Now because we cannot know what God is, but rather what [God] is not, we have no means for considering how God is, but rather how [God] is not (Aquinas 1945, I, 25).

An analysis, by philosopher David Burrell, of the way in which Aquinas used philosophical argument and philosophical expressions indicates "that what holds for the universe cannot hold for [God] as the 'source and goal of all things,' [the phrase with which Thomas defined God]. God's transcendence does not admit of description" (Burrell 1979, 5). At the same time, we can "get an inkling" of God through identifying what cannot be said of God. Paradoxically, the very process of describing transcendence betrays transcendence (Burrell 1979, 7). Analogically, in the sterile language of the neurosciences, the very process of describing the subcortical nonconscious activity of the mammalian and reptilian brains betrays the input of these independent brain systems. Higher processes transform lower processes.

As Aquinas mapped the formal -- that means, rational -- logic of divine affairs, he led us unavoidably to the following assertion:

> . . . the extreme point of the human knowledge of God consists in knowing that God is unknown to us in the sense that [God's] proper being passes beyond all we can

understand of it (*de Potentia* 7.5.14, quoted in Burrell 1979, 174-175).

Thomas' scholastic edifice was more critical than constructive, more analytic than imaginative. It said what could not be said; it could not say what could be said. By "a precise awareness of [the] inadequacy" of language and logic, Thomas displayed a relational discipline which enabled him to "endure," what Burrell calls, "so unknown a God" (Burrell 1979, 58, 67). The logic of the left brain observing, analyzing, and explaining "what God is not" suddenly reveals itself as a whole brain experience of transcendence (cf. Burrell 1979, 71,116).

The spire of Chartres offers a prototypical image in which we can express a sense of the many forces of life without our being diverted from the discovery of Life. Spirelike analysis focuses and directs what we do. Truly, "in the beginning God . . ." (Genesis 1:1) and, "in the beginning Word-Wisdom . . ." (John 1:1). The religious way is a way of inquiry, more accurately, a way of pilgrimage.

Spirelike mentality directs us to identify and to declare, as Aquinas put it, that what is our source is always our good (Aquinas 1945, I, 18). As Burrell puts it, "Once we have grasped how *good* is latent in *being*, we are in a position to make the kind of affirmation which logic prepares us for" (Burrell 1973, 169-170). We become intentional in seeking after that which we already are.

In the language of brain science, cerebral consciousness gives voice to subcortical cognition. The new brain talks about what it gets from the other two brains. The body is in the mind (Johnson 1987), the mind is in the body. Brain is mind, mind is brain.

A Navaho hero-story expressed the same sense of the integrity of reality. "We shall know where we are going when we get there" (Burrell 1973, 73). Or, in Thomas' own words: we are "directed to God as to an end that surpasses the grasp of [our] reason . . . But

TABLE 1 COMPARATIVE OVERVIEW BYZANTINE AND MEDIEVAL CULTURES*

	Byzantine Vision	Medieval Inquiry
Architectural Image:	One Dome	Two Spires
The Working Brain		
brain dominance	relational	rational
mind preference	imaginative	analytic
system preference	visual (icons)	temporal (ideas)
The Work of Theology:		
belief trajectory	manifestation of numinous presence	proclamation of historical claims
source of authority	mystical participation	rational obedience
emphases:		
God as	creating	redeeming
Christ as	triumphant	crucified
Humanity as	participating-in-grace	fallen from grace
Church/Society as	co-equal with open structure	separate spheres with ordered hierarchy
Assessment:		
dominant pattern	abstract-mystical	rational-symbolic
variant patterns	incomplete manifestation deficient proclamation	disturbed proclamation deficient manifestation

* From Ashbrook, 1984c, 261.

the end must first be known by [us] who are to direct [our] thoughts and actions to the end" (Aquinas 1945, I, 6).

CONCLUSION

I draw this analysis of archetypal architecture to a close by a comparative summary of these two ways of knowing God as they are identified in terms of the two ways the brain works: the domelike as discerned in Hagia Sophia and the spirelike as articulated in Chartres (see Table 1).

On the one hand, I have associated the relational dominance of the right hemisphere with the imaginative preference and iconic mode of the Byzantine vision. The central symbol is that of Christ as the Light of the World. On the other hand, I have associated the rational dominance of the left hemisphere with the analytic preference and conceptual mode of Medieval inquiry. Its central symbol is Christ as The Terrible Judge.

Similar contrasts are apparent in theology. There is belief in a manifestation of numinous presence -- world affirmation, if you will, savoring what is. This sense of the numinous is authenticated by mystical participation in a cosmos in which all flows from a creating God. In that universe Christ reigned triumphant and humanity participated in grace. Church and Empire co-existed as co-equals. God could be discerned as surprisingly in the streets as in the sacrament.

On the other hand, there is belief in the proclamation of historical claims -- world transformation, if you will, saving what is to be. This sense of finality was maintained by rational obedience to Authority derived from a redeeming God. In that universe Christ was crucified and humanity had fallen from grace. The spheres of papacy and empire were separate. In the great order of being the spiritual towered over the worldly.

Both the vision of manifestation and the inquiry of proclamation proved precarious -- yet it took a thousand years for the precariousness of each to become obvious!

I think it is no coincidence that under the great dome of St. Sophia we find four huge piers, symbolic of the four corners of the earth and symbolic of the linearity of observing cognition. Nor do I think it is a coincidence that between the towering spires of Chartres we find the great rose window, symbolic of eternity which has no beginning and no ending and symbolic of the all-at-once-ness of our imaginative cognition. Every pattern of belief carries its own complement, even as every strategy of the new brain is derived from a decision made in the old brain as to the nature of the context in which we find ourselves -- is it gracious or is it demonic?

Because of the prototypical-archetypal quality of the dome and the spire, we know that *these are strategies and not Reality*. Whether we enter the realm of the real -- what the Book of Revelation calls the Heavenly City, and New Jerusalem -- through the gate of a rational-explanatory left brain strategy or the gate of a relational-experiential right brain strategy, once there we need all that we are in order to be who we are. Or, perhaps more accurately, we can only enter *any* gate because we already are more than we know ourselves to be and because we intend more than we can ever say.

With the Renaissance, people sought to reestablish control over what they assumed to be "their" world. Measured space replaced infinite space (Zevi 1957, 113-115). Domelike expansiveness has turned into the competition of superdome sports arenas. Spirelike exaltedness has become the excess of skyscrapper aggressiveness. In the transition from sacred spaces as archetypal images of entire cultures, every cultural and social expression, including architecture, has multiplied in exponential ways. Even "The Shopping Mall as Ceremonial Center" (Zepp 1986) threatens to devour the landscape. It provides a center that fails to "center" and a gathering which is not "community." Paradoxically and ironically, more and more buildings are resulting in the world looking "more and more the same." To architectural critic Paul Gapp, we are being engulfed by "The Rise of Generic City" (Gapp 1988).

In the language of theology, we can talk about the Renaissance phenomenon of the mastery of space as the dominance and domination of polytheistic perspectives. Everything goes because nothing matters -- ultimately. Even though the mall is "more than a marketplace," it fails to express the Holy. And in that failure, we now find ourselves at the point where mastery and mystery must be intertwined if we are to survive as human beings on this human planet.

As outward and visible expressions of inward and meaningful experience, architecture articulates the tension between mystery and mastery (Sovik 1973). In describing the tension between "honesty and consecration" in both art and architecture, theologian Paul Tillich insisted that:

> Holy places, holy times, holy acts are necessary as the counterbalance to the secular which tends to cut off our relation to the ultimate . . . and to cover the experience of the holy with the dust of daily life (Tillich 1987, 226).

I suggest that in our time the sense of the ultimate -- the transcendent or the Holy -- is inextricably bound up with the dimension of the genuinely human. Despite its technological advances, contemporary architecture too often ignores the "[h]uman scale, privacy, attunement with nature and respect for historically proven urban values" (Gapp 1988).

We need gathering places that combine "sacred emptiness" and communal utility. Sacred emptiness, in Tillich's terms, represents symbolic space which is "to be filled with the presence of that which cannot be expressed in any finite form" (Tillich 1987, 227), while communal utility serves the technical purpose of making "existence in time and space possible" for us finite creatures (Tillich

1987, 192). From such limited and limiting spaces we can then go forward toward limitless and liberating space.

In the past, *human* dimensions and *human* purposes have become lost in the dissection of *human* life into exclusive spheres of public and private spaces. Architect Philip Bess describes how religious meaning can point the way to architectural renewal, and how architectural renewal can facilitate human renewal. The patterns of our relatedness -- the context in which we are immersed and from which we emerge -- must "promote both communal and personal well-being." From a physical point of view, the city itself needs to "again be seen and built into the symbol of civility and virtue" (Bess 1985). Both "complex individual and societal needs" have to be integrated (Gapp 1988).

We have built our cities without the dimension of transcendence, which means apart from some image of the City of God. Not surprising, then, that life has grown "meaner and uglier" (Bess 1985, 107). The integrated well-being of the whole human family calls for both "spiritual interest and social responsibility" (Zevi 1957, 242), a fullness of reality as the only reality in which we can be the truly human beings that we are, something which no commercial mall can accomplish, magnificent as it is in ordering the chaos of our common sprawl.

The Dome is never an end in itself; the Spire is not the only sure pointer to what matters most, and The Center is never The Holy City of God. In that regard, Tillich articulated the concept of the Protestant Principle. It stands over against making any finite expression ultimate. He defined the principle:

> as the acknowledgment of the majesty of the Divine against every human claim, including every religious claim. From this it follows that no church, and no self-expression of any church, is in itself absolute. There is no absolute unconditional style in any religion (Tillich 1987, 188).

Instead, the domelike, the spirelike, and the centerlike -- in all the imaginative, intentional, and integrative ways we are capable of expressing them -- hold before us archetypal images of what it is for us to stand upright on our feet in a world for which we find ourselves responsible (Genesis 1:28). Only in that transcendent realm at the end of history can the full presence of God become the full presence of humanity. And in that realm, we are told, there is "No temple . . . since the Lord God Almighty and the Lamb [are] themselves the temple" (Revelation 21:22). As Augustine reminds us, the nature of God is comparable to a circle whose center is everywhere and whose circumference is nowhere (Sze [1956] 1959, 30).

In the meantime we go on building, putting into stone the life that is written on our hearts (Jeremiah 31:33).

NOTES

1. In addition to authors cited in the text, I have drawn upon the following: Peter Brown, The Cult of The Saints: Its Rise and Function in Latin Christianity (Chicago: The University of Chicago Press, 1980); George Every, Misunderstandings Between East and West (Richmond, VA: John Knox Press, [1965] 1966); Deno J. Geanakoplos, Byzantine East and Latin West: Two Worlds of Christendom in Middle Ages and Renaissance (Oxford: Basil Blackwell, 1966); Deno J. Geanakoplos, Interaction of The 'Sibling' Byzantine and Western Cultures (New Haven: Yale University Press, 1976); Saint John of Damascus, Writings. Trans. by Frederic H. Chase, Jr. (New York: Fathers of the Church, Inc., 1958); Heinz Kahler, Hagia Sophia. With a chapter on the mosaics by Cyril Mango. Trans. by Ellyn Childs (New York: Praeger Publishers, 1967); R. Krautheimer, Early Christian and Byzantine Architecture (Baltimore: Penguin Books, [1965] 1967); Cyril Mango, Byzantium: The Empire of New Rome (New York: Charles Scribners' Sons, 1980); Thomas F. Mathews, The Early Churches of Constantinople: Architecture and Liturgy (University

Park: The Pennsylvania State University Press, 1971); Thomas F. Mathews, The Byzantine Churches of Istanbul: A Photographic Survey (University Park: The Pennsylvania State University Press, 1976); John Meyendorff, Byzantine Theology: Historical Trends and Doctrinal Themes (New York: Fordham University Press, [1974] 1976); John Meyendorff, Christ in Eastern Christian Thought (Crestwood, NY: St. Vladimir's Seminary Press, 1975); Janet L. Nelson, "Symbols in Context," in The Orthodox Churches and The West, ed. by Derek Baker, 97-119 (Published for the Ecclesiastical History Society Oxford: Basil Blackwell, 1976); Jaroslav Pelikan, The Christian Tradition: A History of The Development of Doctrine. Vol. 1 The Emergence of The Catholic Tradition (100-600); Vol. 2 The Spirit of Eastern Christendom (600-1700) (Chicago: The University of Chicago Press, 1971, 1974); David Talbot Rice, Art of The Byzantine Era (London: Thames and Hudson, 1963); Steven Runciman, Byzantine Style and Civilization (Baltimore: Penguin Books, Inc., 1975); Timothy Ware, The Orthodox Church (Baltimore: Penguin Books, [1963] 1964); Philip Whitting, ed., Byzantium: An Introduction (New York: Harper Torchbooks, [1972] 1973).

2. Evidence and interpretation about personality and emotional correlates of lateralization and damage are controversial. For a different view, see Kinsbourne (1981). I draw on the work of Bear and Fedio (1977) and Mandell (1980). In experiments by Levy, Heller, Barich, and Burton (1983), right-hand subjects with characteristically higher right hemisphere arousal than left hemisphere arousal showed "an optimistic bias, particularly for the left visual field," which sends stimuli to the right hemisphere. For an overview of "Emotional Processes," see Kolb and Whishaw ([1980] 1985, 546-572).

3. In addition to the authors cited in the text, I have drawn on the following: Robert Branner, ed., Chartres Cathedral: Illustrations, Introductory Essays, Documents, Analysis, Criticism (New York: W.W. Norton & Company, 1969); Georges Duby, The Europe of The Cathedrals: 1140-1280, trans. by Stuart Gilbert (Geneva:

Skira, 1966); William Durandus, The Symbolism of Churches and
Church Ornaments. A translation of the first book of the Ration-
ale Divinorum Officiorum, intro. and notes by John Mason Neale
and Benjamin Webb, third edition (London: Gibbings & Com-
pany, 1906); Carolly Erickson, The Medieval Vision: Essays In
History and Perception (New York: Oxford University Press,
1976); Etienne Gilson, History of Christian Philosophy In The
Middle Ages (New York: Random House, 1955); Louis Grodecki,
Gothic Architecture, in collaboration with Anne Prache and
Roland Recht, trans. by I. Mark Paris (New York: Harry N.
Abrams, Inc., [1976] 1977); Raymond Klibansky, "The School of
Chartres," in Twelfth Century Europe And The Foundation of
Modern Society, ed. by Marshall Clagett, Gaines Post, and Robert
Reynolds, 3-14 (Madison, WI: University of Wisconsin Press,
1961); Colin Morris, The Discovery Of The Individual 1050-1200
(New York: Harper Torchbooks, [1972] 1973); Erwin Panofsky,
Gothic Architecture and Scholasticism (New York: Meridan
Books, 1957); Jaroslav Pelikan, The Christian Tradition: A History
Of The Development Of Doctrine. Vol. 3 The Growth Of
Medieval Theology (600-1300) (Chicago: The University of
Chicago Press, 1978); R.W. Southern, The Making Of The Middle
Ages (New Haven: Yale University Press, [1953] 1980).

4. Anselm was more rationalistic than usually perceived. By virtue
of his emphasis on necessary reason in demonstrating faith, he
resisted subordinating reason to faith. Instead, he placed reason
between faith and vision (Fairweather 1970, Anselm, 48, note 8).
Abelard, in contrast, is less rationalistic than on first reading.
Over against his "intransigent confidence in his own reason . . . set
the genuine faith and piety expressed in [his] liturgical poetry"
(Fairweather 1970, 224-225).

5. See Note 2. Levy et al (1983) demonstrated that subjects with
strong right visual field advantage had a pessimistic bias for rating
performance. In personal conversation, she indicated that the left
hemisphere leveled, or neutralized, affect, while weak right hemisphere dominance resulted in a pessimistic biasing. Since spirelike

mentality begins with faith, which suggests a relational right mind process, the correspondence between weak right hemisphere processing, conflictual left and right hemisphere processing in which the vigilant left half struggles to take the lead over the right, and pessimistic tarnishing of experience all contribute to the plausibility of the interpretation.

6. Burrell (1973; 1979) persuasively contrasts the medieval positions of John Duns Scotus' rigidified univocity, or single meaning, of analogous terms and Aquinas' metaphorized analogical usage of language in his shifting the focus from ontological metaphysical objectivity to judgment about logical issues. Instead of the supposed Thomist idiom of "analogy of being," his more usual expression was "analogously speaking" (Burrell 1973, 121).

CHAPTER TWO

IN THE IMAGE AND LIKENESS OF GOD

MALE AND FEMALE

in the image of God...
male and female God created them.
(Genesis 1:27 RSV)

there are no more distinctions between
Jew and Greek,
slave and free,
male and female,
but all of you are one in Christ Jesus.
(Galatian 3:28 JB)

I begin with a personal experience, one which many share. It involves the ways my wife and I drive the car. For years we thought the difficulties were ours alone. Although the difficulties are still ours to cope with, now we recognize these differences are more universal, something basic to how men and women experience "reality" and act on the basis of those perceptions. We are discovering that our genes make more of a difference between us than we suspected.

Here is the situation: On days when the weather is bad -- drenching rain, blanketing snow, or buffeting wind -- she kindly offers to drive me to work on her way to work. Our route brings us down a small grade to the corner of a major intersection. A traffic signal automatically changes from green to yellow to red. At the corner we are confronted with drivers coming toward us -- some cross in front of us as they turn left, some continue toward us as they proceed around the turning cars, and some turn left in the direction we intend to turn. What I describe is ordinary experience -- an intersection and decisions about how to proceed.

One day when she was driving and I was riding, I saw a car barrelling toward us at full speed. I gasped. Fortunately, no collision occurred. However, once the emergency passed, my wife declared, "If you don't like the way I drive, you drive." I felt chastened, and rightly so. From then on I took care *not* to attend to traffic and to let her drive her way. After all, she spent much of her day driving the congested streets of Chicago, and she has not had an accident. My vigilance only endangered both of us.

A few days later she again offered to drive me to work. Since we were still working out a less stressful driving arrangement, I drove and she rode. Again we approached the intersection. Suddenly she gasped. Fortunately, no collision occurred, but once the emergency passed, I though of returning her ultimatum: "If you don't like the way I drive, you drive." If I had, neither of us would likely have ever gotten into a car together again. And *that* would *really* be a problem.

Let me identify what we are recognizing out of such encounters. When she finds herself in a situation of uncertainty -- such as several cars coming at her, slowing down, waiting, or moving ahead -- she slows down. When I find myself in a similar situation of uncertainty -- such as several cars coming at me, slowing down, waiting, or moving ahead -- I speed up.

As we talked about our reactions, we discovered differences in how we perceive reality and how we act on those perceptions. She slows down because she wants to find out what the other drivers will do before she moves. So she waits and gets through safely. I speed up because I want to get out of everybody's way to avoid a traffic jam. So I dart ahead and get through safely. However, when I was riding, I "knew" her hesitancy would result in our being sideswiped, and when she was riding, she "knew" my impulsivity would result in our being sideswiped. As long as we drove separately, we were safe. The problem came when we drove together. *Then* there could be a collision!

From Personal Stress to Universal Differences

I describe this minor incident for a reason. It personalizes exchanges couples have about -- going on vacation, shopping, fixing the house, doing the laundry, getting together with families, going to church, being active in the community, opening and closing windows in the bedroom, engaging in sexual intercourse, doing Christmas cards. It illustrates differences men and women generally have over issues like: what interests them on radio or television; how they shop; how they negotiate differences; how they evaluate workshops; how they work in the church; how they teach a class; how they administer a parish.

My wife and I even differ as to the situation I have described -- while acknowledging my point about our differences, she feels this example applies more to driving than to gender, and I am convinced it applies more to gender than simply to driving. We even differ about our differences! She focuses more on what is specific; I focus more on what is general -- at least much of the time.

Test my point. Take any strange situation involving you and your spouse or a friend of the opposite sex. I say "strange" because only a strange situation stresses us to the point of reacting in terms of our basic survival strategies: our instinctual behavior (the reptilian mind) which influences the emotional meaning of the situation (the mammalian mind) and determines how we handle the threat (the rational mind). While my interpretation may be simplistic, in the groups to which I speak from 2/3rds to 3/4ths of the people report a dynamic similar to the one I describe between my wife and me at the intersection.

> Men respond to one reality and women to another --
> *and neither of us realizes we are dealing with different*
> *realities.* Even though the elements in the picture are
> the same, our experiences of the picture, which means

the significance of meaning of the picture, generate contrasting responses, and under stress, conflicting responses.

I recognize that men differ as much from each other -- and more so in many instances -- than any particular man differs from any particular woman. Similarly, women differ as much from each other -- and more so in many instances -- than any particular women differs from any particular man. As psychiatrist Harry Stack Sullivan said, we are more simply human than otherwise.

Even so, I contend that what is true in little ways is equally true in larger ways. We approach the crossroads of our lives as though we each see, sense, select, and respond in the same way to the same reality. In Chapter Five on epistemology, I describe a basic shift in cognition from fixed features to experiential realism. I link that shift to increased knowledge of the brain. Here I go further. I submit that the new paradiam of knowledge -- and, therefore, a new paradigm of what constitutes reality -- arises because men and women do not see, do not sense, do not select, and do not respond in the same way to the same reality.

I would agree that we can identify a great deal of ordinary commonality -- a street, a church, our home, our children, our country, the Bible, the stars. In addition, as we grow accustomed to our separate "realities," the more these differences recede. With age women and men become more androgynous. Couples seem to think alike. In truth, what constitutes truth requires the experiences of all peoples in all places.

But, in strange situations, our mind experiences anxiety and our body reacts with stress. Our autonomic (limbic) and instinctual (reptilian) systems take over. In addition to our socialized roles, we confront different realities; we experience different demands; we select different strategies to cope with different situations. I submit gender differences make a difference that *is* a difference!

Experience and Epistemology

Underneath ideologies about patriarchy, feminism, and exclusive versus inclusive language lies the issue of epistemology: "how" do we "know;" and based on that way of knowing, "what" do we know? What we take to be knowledge comes from experience.

Historically, many men have expressed reservation about experience. It is reflected in their minimizing "women's intuition." They claim that an experiential approach to knowledge easily falls into the trap of subjective bias. As a check on individual distortion, therefore, they approach issues as objectivity as possible. They are suspicious of anything "subjective."

In contrast, most women prize experience. Feminist thinkers criticize male-valued objectivity as "inherently distorting." It inverts some of life's "real regularities" (Harding and Hintikka 1983, x; Bynum, Harrell, and Richman 1986, 13). "Women's Ways of Knowing," to use the title of a recent book (Belenky et al 1986), involve experiential participation. Without that, what is known distorts what is to be known. They are suspicious of anything "objective."

Philosopher Jane Flax insists that "a feminist theory of knowledge" begins "by examining how and why the dilemmas projected onto the world as the 'human condition' in fact have their social roots in a virtually universal kind of masculine experience. The apparently irresolvable dualisms of subject-object, mind-body, inner-outer, reason-sense reflect real but repressed dilemmas originating in masculine infantile experience of the sexual division of labor" (Harding and Hintikka 1983, xviii; Flax 1983, 269-270).

My editorial consultant Barbara Stinchcombe added at this point in the manuscript:

> The oldest ongoing battle in the world is the one between the sexes. They are always in turmoil. I don't know if "the sexual division of labor" was as significant

as women's ability to bear children -- to visibly create a human being. It was potency and power, which men could only equal by engaging in war, which was a symbolic means of control over the universe joined to a likewise real control over life and death, which women handled naturally.

It must have been an awesome thing for early man to see his mate give birth -- to create another like herself or himself and survive. In any society it is a feat that cannot be surpassed -- it can however be diminished in significance by subjugating the women who have this power of say over creativity.

A female oriented epistemology insists upon experience; a male oriented epistemology rejects experience.

Yet even this clash over "experience," I suggest, reflects different realities to which "experience" refers. Experience is not the same for men and women. Thus, even what constitutes knowledge differs in some respects because its origins differ in basic respects.

I take a further step before returning to a more detailed analysis of the issue:

> *if* how men and women know -- and know that they know -- differs, then how men and women know God -- and know that they know God -- must differ also.

Ultimate reality and ordinary reality make up the same reality of what matters most to our being the human beings that we are. Breath and dust, I insist, are one reality -- the brain as mind and the mind as brain. God is God of all, yet men and women experience, and express, that reality differently. *And that difference makes a basic difference in the lives we live.*

Having stated my conclusion as strongly as I can, let me share the process by which I have arrived at such a conviction.

Of course being married and raising a family of one boy and three girls have contributed to my conviction that the difference between men and women makes a difference. Even so, this personal history did not take on compelling power *until* other evidence accumulated. Women students and women colleagues have pressed me about my patriarchial bias, even when I have not exhibited more objectionable forms of male chauvinism. As I have tried to make sense of their sensitivity and my insensitivity, I have begun to see more through their eyes. I am seeing that the pattern of oppression, the teeter-totter of dominance and submission, is both subtle and rampant, like Nasrudin's donkeys.

Socialization of Gender

The socialization of gender *is* clear -- we *do* treat boys and girls differently.

The politicization of power *is* rampant -- we *do* reward men and women differently, even for the same efforts.

The stereotyping of role possibilities *is* a fact -- there are some things which mosı men simply *do not do* and some things which most women simply *do not do*.

Knowledge in the "hard" physical sciences, no less than in the "soft" human sciences, has come from, what one interpreter calls, "distinctive and often perverse masculine understandings of only masculine social experience" (Harding and Hintikka 1983, xiii) -- men create compartments of experience and women emphasize connections in experience (Bynum, Harrell, and Richman 1986; Bynum 1987).

The Reader's Digest carried an article entitled "5 Sex Secrets Women Wish Their Husbands Knew" (McCoy 1988, 91-94). The author reports that some husbands are puzzled that their wives find it hard to be enthusiastic and passionate in bed *after* an exchange of hurtful words, inattentiveness, and criticism. Husbands tend to live in separate spaces, while wives experience the whole house.

For instance, a forty-three year old man, who had been married for 24 years, said that for him, "Sex can be a comfort after a rotten day. Why can't a woman see sex as its own moment in time -- and forget what's gone before?" But according to sociologist Lynn Atwater, "Women see everything in their lives as interconnected. Men tend to compartmentalize, feeling that stressful time can be parked mentally and separated from sexual actions." In the words of sex researcher Virginia Johnson Masters, "Sexuality and affection *can't* be compartmentalized. Good sex is a continuum of closeness and affection."

Of course, whether sex is connected with closeness is a matter of degree. Yet that small degree of difference makes a difference to both parties. The couple which does not understand that difference finds itself in trouble, partially satisfied, partially frustrated, continually uncertain. The couple which does understand that difference finds itself more fully satisfied, less often frustrated, and increasingly confident in their relationship. Each partner realizes the other comes at sexuality and affection slightly differently. Neither approach is better or worse than the other, only different.

I shift from sex to science. As a system of beliefs, science has acquired a gender -- what professor of mathematics and humanities Evelyn Fox Keller refers to as "a 'genderization of' science" (Keller 1983, 188). By that she means, science itself has reflected masculine values rather than more broadly human values. In an analogous way, theology, as a system of beliefs, has acquired a gender -- what amounts to "a genderization of theology." By that I mean, theology itself has reflected masculine values rather than more broadly human values. Nothing in life, no matter how trivial or important, has escaped the acquisition of gender identification.

Feminist thinkers remind us that we all live under "genderization." At its worst, genderization arises from oppressive patriarchy; at its best, it appears with constricting sexism. Because childrearing experiences tend to "associate the affective and cognitive posture of objectification with [the] masculine . . . [and] all [other] processes which involve a blurring of the boundary between subject and object . . . with the feminine," "truth itself has become genderized" (Keller 1983, 197-198).

I hear that criticism and I learn from it. But my own conviction about the origin and support of genderizing, with its distortion of full human life, comes more from brain research than from feminist thinkers. They put my conviction about gender differences into the larger social context where people politicize values. Nevertheless, I think biological differences influence that sexist distortion as do historical forces.

Gender Predisposition and Neuropsychological Effects

In my view, distortions of human values arise from genetic predispositions and their resulting neuropsychological consequences. Because the brains of men and women differ in certain basic features, we experience different experiences, we listen with different ears, we speak in different voices, we see with different eyes, we feel with different viscera, we respond with different values. In short, we make or interpret reality in different ways. While my concerns are similar to feminists, I have travelled a different route. It is that route which I describe.

First, I report on evidence about the different brain organizations of men and women. Then, I relate those differences to our understanding of God, what it means to be created in the image of God, and the difference that makes in the ways we believe and behave. Finally, I qualify these stark statements with other evidence which suggests the differences may relate more to the rate of maturation than to specific gender predisposition. I must say, however, that despite the ambiguity of maturation and despite the prevalence of patriarchy, I remain convinced that an understanding of the biological origins of these differences will make us all more humane than we might otherwise be.

Some evidence is certain; other controversial (McGlone 1980; Goy and McEwen 1980; Kolb and Whishaw [1980] 1985, 363-372; Springer and Deutsch [1981] 1985, 175-185). In the early 1970s researchers such as Eleanor Emmons Maccoby and Carol Nagy Jacklin (1974) minimized sex differences; in the early 1980s others like Carol Gilligan ([1982] 1983) were reendorsing sex differences (Bynum, Harrell, and Richman 1986, 12-13). One investigator summarized the literature on gender as "rife with inconsistencies" (Bryden 1982, 238).

What we conclude must be taken with caution. Differences have proven to be of such modest proportions and to involve such complex variables that there can be more difference between any two males or any two females than between any particular male and any particular female (Hyde 1981). The most predictive use of the gender variable requires us to put gender in context, that is, what specific conditions influence the display of gender related behavior (Deaux and Major 1987).

What is known empirically about the similarities and differences in the brains of men and women?

Genetic-Hormonal Origins

As early as the sixth week of pregnancy the crucial crystallization of sexual differentiation occurs (Benderly 1987, 14). Until that "moment" the embryo is undifferentiated, neither female nor male; it simply is "human potentiality." More suggestive is the fact that "the basic plan of the mammalian organism is female and stays that way unless told to be otherwise by masculine hormones" (Konner [1982] 1983, 122). Then fetal androgens begin "organizing" the neuroanatomy of behavior for future reproductive activity (Hopson 1984, 70-73; Springer and Deutsch [1981] 1985, 180-181). These androgens "tune" certain cells to the hormones which will flood the body at puberty. Specifically, the androgen "tuning" suppresses the capacity for monthly cycling in males (Benderly 1987, 17-18).

As birth approaches, the masculinizing hormones, primarily testosterone, have so affected the development of the brain that a trained observer, "holding a microscope slide [of the hypothalamus] up to the light, can tell the sex of the brain with the naked eye" (Konner [1982] 1983, 125-126, 115ff). We can sense the significance of this prebirth difference in the fact that the hypothalamus acts as "an all-powerful liaison between brain and body." It serves as "a master control center for basic drives and visceral functions in the brain's core" (Hooper and Teresi [1986] 1987, 35, 146). Here is the region, along with the limbic system, which plays a primary role "in courtship, sex, maternal behavior, and violence" (Konner [1982] 1983, 117).

From that early differentiation, we become vulnerable in different ways. Psychiatrist Pierre Flor-Henry (1983), for instance, claims that our different brain organizations put us at risk for different kinds of mental illnesses (cited in Benderly 1987, 245). These illnesses are "usually triggered" in our "weaker" hemispheres. Male brains become more vulnerable to malfunctions linked with the left hemisphere -- "autism, schizophrenia, and psychopathy." Female brains exhibit an earlier maturation of the left hemisphere and are subject more to mood disorders controlled by the right hemisphere. Boys are more likely than girls to experience learning disorders and behavioral restlessness.

The differences in vulnerability are positive as well. Physically, girls mature earlier than boys (Kolb and Whishaw [1980] 1985, 370-371). This includes their capacity for language. They talk earlier; they rely more on verbal skills in solving problems, including nonverbal problems such as spatial tasks; they engage in quieter physical activity. In other words, a large percentage of behavior problems in school would be eliminated if boys started two years later than girls. The left hemisphere in girls develops more rapidly than in boys. One consequence is that girls -- generally -- play school more often and longer than boys.

In contrast, the right hemisphere in boys matures earlier than in girls. Boys rely more on physical and spatial perception in engaging the world. They learn more readily by moving around than by talking things through. One consequence is that boys -- generally -- race motor cars and build with blocks more often and longer than girls.

I speculate about the long term effects of early and late maturing of language.

Early Maturers (in language)

Because of the earlier development of the left hemisphere, both hemispheres tend to handle information in similar ways. The left brain processes nonverbal information as well as verbal; the right brain uses verbal strategies as well as nonverbal strategies. There is less division of labor, less specialization between what one half does and what the other half does. The information exchanged between them, thereby, tends to be redundant.

In technical terms, the result is known as weak asymmetry, a more equal distribution of language and perception across both hemispheres (Kolb and Whishaw [1980] 1985, 370-371; Springer and Deutsch [1981] 1985, 183-184). Specialized functions still can be discerned, that is, the left half is more capable of using analytical strategies and the right half is more capable of responding globally, but the tendency is secondary to the similarity -- at least in early maturers (Waber 1976). Each hemisphere functions as a generalist instead of a specialist (Blakeslee 1980, 99-101).

The difference between strong and weak asymmetry, however, is less an absolute fact and more a "dynamic" phenomenon (Martin and Voorhies 1975; Kimura 1985). We are dealing with a continuum of "maleness" and "femaleness." I think of the difference between the brains of male and female as gender related, not gender specific. Evidence suggests several types of brain organization, not two. And these patterns most likely differ at different periods in life (Kimura 1985).

Biopsychologist Jerre Levy (1980b, 367-371) summarizes the implications of that mixture of verbal and nonverbal information in hemisphere organization. People with weak asymmetry, usually female, are more connected with the actual situation in which they find themselves, field dependent to use the technical phrase, and more sensitive to the context, especially its interpersonal nuances. Rather than responding to features of the environment which allow for formal and abstract structures, these individuals respond to subtle experiential clues which interfere with the abstraction process.

Because the two brains are so intimately connected, weak asymmetry facilitates integrating details and nuances of the environment. Perhaps that explains, in part, why a right brain quality like intuition is more prevalent in women (Benderly 1987, 256). At the same time, bilateral distribution of functions creates a liability. The person is less able to hone in on a few details relevant to a crystallized pattern.

In school, early maturers tend to develop better reading skills and give evidence of verbal fluency. In terms of cultural stereotypes, girls enter the world talking and do not stop. They tend to approach situations in terms of sounds, words, and hearing, even as they respond "slightly more eagerly to faces" than boys (Benderly 1987, 248-249). In the early grades girls outscore boys. However, they give evidence of less mathematical reasoning. It is speculated that difficulty in mathematical reasoning occurs because the abstract denotative aspect of the task includes none of the metalinguistic processing of tone and affect to which girls are so attuned.

Later Maturers (in language)

Later maturers of language, according to Levy, show an extreme separation between their verbal skills and their nonverbal abilities.

Each hemisphere specializes in either the rational or relational strategy. The right half handles perceptual information; the left half conceptual information. Instead of each hemisphere being a generalist, as is true of early maturers, each half functions as a specialist. This can lead to such questions as "which is more important -- the sun or the moon," the left hand or the right hand, the right hemisphere or the left hemisphere? Even more, specialization increases the incidence of developmental disorders associated with possible left hemisphere dysfunction (Benderly 1987, 277-278).

The result is a certain independence, or distance, from the environment. One is selectively inattentive -- or insensitive, as the case might be -- to what is going on. Technically, this is called field independence (Witkin and Goodenough 1981, 67). The person becomes adept at extricating abstract features from the environment. These features are relevant to spatial organization and logical structure. In school, later maturers are better in verbal reasoning and formal language. They are more geared to objects and sight than to people and listening (Benderly 1987, 248-249). Because they have already generated an abstract map, they have difficulty processing experiential representations which closely resemble original perceptions. Instead of the territory, they use the map. And, as the saying goes: the map is not the territory (Korzybski 1933).

Gender Related

As with Nasrudin smuggling donkeys, these differences are so obvious we tend to overlook them. Much of the time men and women "attend to different aspects of the same event" (Benderly 1987, 248).

For instance, what happens when a couple gets lost on a trip? The husband tends to keep on driving; convinced he will figure out where they are without having to ask. The wife urges him to stop and ask for help; or else she pores over a map trying to make sense of what she can see on paper. Basically, the man moves around, that is his way of coping with uncertainty; the woman talks, that is her way of coping with uncertainty. Occasionally, they blow up. The way each copes annoys the other.

In brief, men tend to attend to the physical world and its abstract features; women to the social world and its tangible aspects. Women handle varied conditions better, while men zero in on simplified features. Males process images and shapes more easily than females, and visual perception is crucial in the physical world. The fact that females process sounds and language more easily (Coltheart, Hull, and Slater 1975) tends to impede their spatial capacities and strengthen their interpersonal skills (Kolb and Whishaw [1980] 1985, 372).

Spatial ability is one of the clearest differences. A figure drawing used to diagnose frontal lobe disease elicited stylistic differences in normal subjects (Waber 1979, 172-176). The children were instructed to copy the figure by using colored pencils, in a standard order. Based on their performance researchers identified copying strategies.

At age five, girls reproduced more parts of the design more accurately than boys. In addition, they drew more discrete parts of the picture. Boys reproduced more of the external features. By age 11, the differences in accuracy or organization had disappeared. However, the use of colored pencils showed different strategies for accomplishing the same task. The males drew their figures "in long, sweeping, continuous lines, while females drew theirs part by part." By age 13, these stylistic differences had disappeared also.

Despite their disappearance many people experience such stylistic differences -- take the matter of planning a vacation, for instance.

A man says, "Let's take a vacation." With that, he has a trip projected. The wife dampens his excitement by details she claims have to be attended to before they can take off: where will they go, who will make the reservations, how will they get there, what about stopping the daily newspaper, will the post office hold the mail? The details seem endless. As she focuses on the practicalities, he feels thwarted.

The woman, in turn, reacts to her husband's impulsivity. How can he ignore the practical issues: where will they go, can they get reservations, what about cleaning the kitchen and straightening up the bedroom, what clothes do they have, who will take care of the cat?

She attends to the details *in order to go*; he attends to the destination *in order to get there*. Each wants the vacation, yet each experiences the other's reaction as a problem.

As I have indicated, stylistic differences tend to disappear by adulthood. Yet with puberty the differences between the sexes become blatant. By then, the effects of socialization have become established. Despite great overlap between men and women in most aspects of experience, differences are not only discernible, they are obvious (McGlone 1980).

Developmental Differences

However, women researchers and feminist critics have identified more subtle differences.

For instance, what is understood as normal psychosocial development has come under scrutiny. Traditionally, Sigmund Freud focused upon the competition between the father and son for the wife/mother as the favored woman in their lives. Today, psychoanalyst Nancy Chodorow ([1978] 1979) and psychologist Jean Baker Miller ([1976] 1986), among others (Glaz 1987), reject that paradigm of competition for the more humane and human pattern of cooperation. Cooperation arises from the bonding of mother and infant.

Furthermore, Erik Erikson's theory of human development has identified a sequence of psychosocial features. From an initial experience of trust versus mistrust, there emerge stages of autonomy versus shame and doubt, initiative versus guilt, industry versus inferiority, identity versus ego diffusion, intimacy versus isolation, generativity versus stagnation, and ego integrity versus despair. Again, the conventional paradigm has been called into question. Girls develop in a different way. For them, identity and intimacy are simultaneous, not sequential. Autonomy is never separated from attachment. The stages blend self and others without giving priority to one over the other.

For over a decade, Carol Gilligan ([1982] 1983) worked with Lawrence Kohlberg's theory of moral development, based on the work of Jean Piaget in cognition. She began to discern different responses between men and women in moral decision-making. Gilligan concluded that male socialization included few experiences of care for, and nurture of, others, resulting in a male tendency to neglect the care and responsibility of others. Girls, in contrast, experienced the bonding of identity-and-intimacy in ways which enhanced concern with responsibility and care for others. Boys become persons by separating from the mother and distinguishing themselves from others; girls become persons by connecting with the mother and affiliating with others.

Because of these differences in child-rearing, adult men tend to come at moral issues in terms of abstract principles and matters of justice. Adult women, in contrast, tend to deal with moral issues in terms of concrete concerns for everyone involved and matters of ongoing care.

Studies such as Gilligan's provide evidence that early maturers are more likely to be sensitive to the context in which they find themselves, to take in more of the interpersonal complexity, and to avoid setting people against each other. Late maturers, when and if they are boys, are more likely to be insensitive to the context, simplify its complexity, and place its various aspects into sharper categories of "right" and "wrong," "good" and "bad," or "important" and "unimportant." This may reflect socialization pressure and so be a protective device until they can get outside the house where their identity can be freer to establish itself as male.

Again editorial consultant Stinchcombe responds at length to the text:

> Society encourages girls to learn to want to bear children, to expect to bear children. It wants boys to be toughened for survival in the world so as to become heads of family and support the next generation. One of the upsets about women's liberation has been the fear that maybe the women will just give up child bearing -- watch the media, read the articles -- consider the latent messages: If you're not married by 30, you'll be an old maid. Women who bear children before 30 have a lower incidence of breast cancer. There are lots of different reasons society trashes women's efforts, but one outstanding one is fear they may just not bear children anymore. You could even argue that the "break throughs" in artificial insemination and laboratory births are perhaps a very real assurance to a male dominated science that they can create the next generation on their own terms -- science fiction? It all depends.

It is apparent men and women deal with life differently (Kolb and Whishaw [1980] 1985, 372). Perhaps only a male would identify the differences as sharply as I do, but in the feminist criticisms such differences are linked with gender contrast. I distinguish between "feminine" and "masculine" in a way that relates these qualities to gender without restricting them to either sex. The qualities are gender related without being gender specific. That means, any woman may exhibit less of a feminine quality than a particular man, and any man may exhibit less of a masculine quality than a particular woman. Even so, the distinctions arise because of gender predispositions, many of which have become laden with positive and negative valuation.

Gender Qualities and Dendritic Density

Feminine qualities reflect more tolerance of ambiguity and mystery, while masculine qualities focus on clear structures and definite decisions. The feminine exhibits more respect for nonrational contrasts, whereas the masculine demands logical reasons. The feminine trusts the intuitive, while the masculine depends more upon authority. The feminine deals more openly with feelings, while the masculine attends to analysis. The feminine exhibits a broad range of interests, whereas the masculine tends toward specialized interests. In contrast to a more stabilized reality for men, women experience reality as more fluid.

I relate such differences to how our brains are wired neurologically and how hormones affect development. Information is processed through a neuronal structure of nerve cells (Kolb and Whishaw [1980] 1985, 32-54). These cells consist of a nucleus, a single axonal trunk, and branching offshoots known as dendrites. Researcher Marian Diamond compares the palm of her hand to the cell body and her fingers to the dendrites (Hopson 1984, 70). The dendrites fan out to connect with other dendrites so that the nucleus can process the information and send it on by means of its axon.

Studies suggest that, as a group, women have denser dendritic structures than men. This is an inference based on data from both humans and rats. It is most apparent in terms of the left hemisphere and the left side of the hippocampus in experiments with rats (Springer and Deutsch [1981] 1985, 212-213; Hopson 1984, 73). While both hippocampi are crucial for normal memory, the left contributes more to verbal material and the right, which is larger in male rats, is more important in visual and spatial memory (Kolb and Whishaw [1980] 1985, 478-488). During pregnancy, the cortex of female rats grows larger. Diamond believes this phenomenon "would make sense, in evolutionary terms, for the female to be at her optimum behavioral capacity during and after pregnancy . . . [helping] her to prepare for and protect her young".

(Hopson 1984, 73). Although the numerous reports of large differences between the sexes in both the neocortex and hypothalamus of rats have not yet been substantiated in humans, "[t]here is no reason to believe that similar differences are not present in humans" (Kolb and Whishaw [1980] 1985, 359).

I infer that the branching neural network of women has more interconnections than that of men. It is as though men have neuronal trees, while women have neuronal bushes. A primary consequence of these differences comes with the rapidity and certainty of what each person knows. Men tend to arrive at conclusions faster, whereas women tend to come to conclusions more slowly (Kolb and Whishaw [1980] 1985, 365).

I have learned that when I really want to know what my wife thinks about something, I present the matter and wait -- patiently -- for twenty-four hours. Then she tells me what she thinks, based on an inner sifting of complex data. I have difficulty waiting yet have learned its value.

The difference, I believe, is related to dendritic density. I have fewer branches and more trunks which carry information; she has more branches and fewer trunks which carry information. Thus, I tend to jump to conclusions, and she tends to consider alternatives. Over time, neither way is better. Each has its strengths; each its weakness. When life goes well, we tango; under stress, we tangle.

According to anthropologist Melvin Konner, two gender patterns are universal. Males tend toward aggression and females tend toward affiliation. Boys show greater egoism and/or aggression than girls. The result, he concludes, is that in terms of averages, the world would be safer if the weapon systems were controlled by the average female rather than the average male (Konner [1982] 1983, 126). In fact, if the average female was in charge, there would be fewer weapon systems even needing to be controlled.

Implications For Belief

While the above has interest for the differing psychologies of men and women, you may ask: what relevance does this have to theology and the ways people believe?

Our brains are double as I describe more fully in the following chapters. The two halves divide the labor and handle information differently. The left brain proceeds item-by-item and step-by-step. This narrow logical style admits only "a few members to any one category" and attends "to detail in small differences" (Kinsbourne 1982). It observes, organizes, and explains things systematically. It is always "on alert," constantly vigilant, isolating and mastering what needs to be taken into account in accomplishing conscious purposes. In short, it explains what it observes in a rational way.

In contrast, the right brain functions all-at-once and by leaps of imagination. This broad integrative style groups "a wide variety of similar objects or concepts together, paying little attention to detail or difference" (Kinsbourne 1982). It creates a web of connections which blurs differences and emphasizes similarities. It interacts constantly with the environment, responding without labeling. In short, it expresses the felt-meaning of what is happening.

In summary, then, the left brain explains things logically. The right brain experiences imaginatively. These patterns make the left brain vigilant and the right brain responsive. Neither functions alone. Each depends on what the other contributes. Together, they make for a unified consciousness and integrated behavior.

Researcher Doreen Kimura (1985) has compared brain organization in men and women. Speech production and hand movement for women primarily involves the left front hemisphere, while for men they involve the whole left hemisphere. For both functions, therefore, the sexes differ. Women's brain organization is more focal.

I infer from these differences that women are more intentional or conscious of what they say and how they use their hands. Male speech and hand use are more a blend of sensory input and motor output. This suggests to me why I tend to talk out loud to find out what I think, while my wife tends to think things through and then speak what she has thought. When she talks, she knows what she is going to say, at least much of the time.

In terms of other verbal tasks, however, the front left hemisphere of both men and women is involved. These include naming words which begin with certain letters. In addition it includes describing appropriate social behavior.

More significantly, a difference is found in the ways women and men define words (Kimura 1985).

> For men, the process is confined to their whole left hemisphere. The result of the "naming" and "analyzing" processes makes the meaning of words more precise and, if you will allow this generalization, more conceptual. This, we now know, accompanies the later maturation of language and the specialization of the two hemispheres.

> For women, however, both hemispheres are involved in word definitions. In fact, both front and back parts of both hemispheres are involved. The effect is evident in the fact that the source for women's understanding is more diffuse, less conceptual, less dependent upon exact dictionary definitions and more dependent on experiential processes.

These differences help me understand the importance of "experience" in "women's ways of knowing" (Belenky et al 1986).

Religious Experiences

Elsewhere I have shown (Ashbrook 1984b; 1984c) that traditional patterns of belief parallel the two processes of rational explanation and relational experience. Generally, people have expressed their perception of God in one of two ways: either a hermeneutics of proclamation or a phenomenology of manifestation (Ricouer 1978; Tracy 1981).

Proclamation interprets what has been experienced in historical events, such as Exodus and Easter. It makes the significance of life explicit. This reflects the logic of the left brain. Deliberate intention is required to make right what is real. Proclamation is "Word" oriented in that we are to hear the truth and are to act on the basis of it: "Hear, O Israel . . ." and "You have heard it said . . . but I say unto you . . ." This theology emphasizes redemption, based upon instructions and imperatives. We are obedient to what is urgently right.

Manifestation, in contrast, expresses the rhythmic processes of the natural order. It elicits wonder and awe for which no words are adequate. This reflects the intuition of the right brain. Manifestation is object oriented in that it is more experienced than expressed. "The heavens declare the glory of God, and the firmament showeth God's handiwork" (Psalm 19:1). This theology emphasizes creation, the celebration of God's presence everywhere and in everything. We trust what is ultimately real.

Now I connect the brain with belief in terms of gender. Pastoral psychologist David Pierce developed an empirical way to understand how people process religious experience (Pierce 1986). He presented subjects with two cognitive approaches to biblical material -- one analytic and the other imagistic.

With 104 students, half women and half men, from five seminaries, he took a color photograph of Rembrandt's painting titled "Storm on the Sea of Galilee" and gave them the following instructions: "Your task is to take a few minutes to experience the painting as much as possible and then write [down] what you perceive as you look at the painting." He also gave them the passage of Jesus and the disciples caught in the storm, as described in Luke 8:22-25, and instructed them to: "Meditate on the following scripture for a few minutes and then write [down] the titles of sermons which you think would clearly indicate important perceptions from the passage."

This use of picture and text allowed for a wide range of ideas and perceptions. He clustered the responses according to major themes, which accounted for 92% of the responses, and identified themes as follows: 1) overwhelming experiences, 2) ongoing presence of God, 3) dependency on Christ, 4) calmness in the storm, 5) violent struggle, 6) test of faith, 7) attempting to stay in control, 8) power of God, 9) peaceful light, and 10) obedience to Christ. Using these themes, students then compared each theme with each of the other themes in a paired comparison format designed to indicate how similar or dissimilar they thought each pair of themes was.

Three distinct dimensions emerged.

> *Dimension I*: One pole correlated with the themes "test of faith," "obedience to Christ," and "overwhelming experiences." Compared to the other themes, these three emphasized the cost of discipleship, or the natural consequence of being part of the group sent by Jesus to the other side of the lake. Thus, for this pole, students used the central theme of being obedient to Christ to organize their responses.

> By contrast, the themes representing the other end of the dimension were "peaceful light," "calmness in the storm," and "crossing over." This cluster related to the blessings of God in the midst of a trial. When taken alone, the themes of "peaceful light" and "calmness in the storm" reflect a sense of the pervasive presence and

power of God. When, however, "crossing over" was chosen as more important than the themes "power of God" and "ongoing presence of God," crossing to the other side was most likely seen as a positive outcome, or blessing, which was made possible by the paradoxical situation of experiencing a peaceful light and a calmness in a raging storm.

This dimension (COST/BLESSING) represents a continuum between the cost of discipleship at one end of the scale and the blessings of God at the other end. The dimension seems to correspond to a theology of the cross as one pole and to a theology of glory as the other. In other words, the dimension distinguished between being obedient, with a sense of integrity, or having trust, with a sense of involvement.

Pierce noted that this dimension paralleled the polishing effect of the right brain in which things are seen to be better than they are, and the tarnishing effect of the left brain in which things are perceived to be worse than they are.

On the BLESSING side, the themes reflected imperturbability. Given the storm and the danger, the idea of "crossing over in the presence of a peaceful light and calmness" clearly underestimates the negative circumstances. In fact, it takes a leap of imagination, rather than a rational explanation, to connect "crossing over" in a life-threatening storm with "peaceful light" and "calmness." Such a relaxed response, reflecting right brain process which smoothes over the rough and shines up the dark (Ashbrook 1984c, 48), defined this pole of the dimension.

Tarnishing has been linked with the left brain. It involves a "dulling or spoiling or tainting of what is" (Ashbrook 1984c, 43). When extreme, tarnishing leads to a sense of being on the verge of disaster. The COST side of the dimension showed that reaction. Its main ideas were: "overwhelming experiences," while being "obedient to Christ," during "a test of faith." Together, the themes emphasize a catastrophic view of the situation. Every theme which hinted at the power, presence, action, or effect of God correlated negatively with this pole of the dimension.

In summary, the BLESSING pole of the dimension is identified with the need for the disciples to be involved with the manifestation of God's provision of peace, calm and getting across the lake. The COST pole is related to the call for integrity through obedience. Thus, Pierce associated a theology of proclamation, the call for loyal obedience, and left brain process. Similarly, he connected a theology of manifestation, the call for trusting dependence, and right brain process.

The polar dimension of COST versus BLESSING supports my suggestion of how God acts in the world in light of the two ways the hemispheres work.

> *Dimension II*: Pierce labelled the second dimension IN-STRUMENTAL versus RELATIONAL. The IN-STRUMENTAL pole was represented by the themes: "attempting to stay in control," "holding on for life," and "violent struggle." These suggested the instrumental efforts of the disciples to survive rather than an intrinsic relationship with God. The themes of "obedience to Christ" and "dependency on Christ" correlated negatively with this pole. The pattern is one of control in the midst of tension.

> The other end of the dimension was RELATIONAL. Two themes indicated a symbolic relationship with nature, that is, peaceful light in the midst of danger, and a paradoxical calmness in the storm. The other three themes -- namely, "obedience to Christ," "ongoing presence of God," and "dependency on Christ" -- each indicated an intimate link between the divine and the

human. In contrast to the struggle for survival, this pole suggested an assurance of well-being.

We know that left brain process is deliberate, controlled, convergent. The theme of "attempt to stay in control" was the most important one for the INSTRUMENTAL pole. When combined with the next most important theme, "holding on for life," the need for deliberate and conscious control is obvious. Each of the themes implies danger and focuses only on the disciples themselves, thereby ignoring awareness of a relationship with God or Jesus.

By contrast, right brain process is immediate, imaginative, divergent. The theme of "peaceful light" emerged as the most important for the RELATIONAL pole. Other themes included calmness in the storm and a personal relationship with Christ and God. There was an absence of any instrumental response.

> *Dimension III*: Pierce called the third, and last, dimension HUMAN EFFORTS versus DIVINE POWER. Two themes represented the HUMAN EFFORTS pole: "crossing over" and "violent struggle." Getting across the lake was primary. When that was associated with violent struggle, the efforts of the disciples lacked reference to any reality other than their own power. This pattern is consistent with left brain process and limbic arousal. We are on our own and under pressure to make it on our own.

In contrast, the themes of "power of God," "calmness in the storm," and "ongoing presence of God" represented the pole of DIVINE POWER. God was seen as actively involved in the storm. There is no hint of human effort or human responsibility. The themes of power, calmness, presence, and light reflect a right brain way of believing, which, I suggest, is derived from the limbic activity of relaxing in the face of a gracious or benevolent environment.

In summary, seminary students were asked to process material depicting Jesus and the disciples crossing the sea of Galilee. Three polar dimensions emerged: COST/BLESSING, which appeared to parallel the polishing and the tarnishing effects of right and left brain attributes; INSTRUMENTAL/RELATIONAL, which reflected the relational and the rational strategies of the right and left brains, respectively; and HUMAN EFFORTS/DIVINE POWER, which distinguished the explanation of the left brain and the imagination of the right brain. These dimensions reflected both the analytic process of the text and the imagistic process of the painting. The dimensions were polar. Students used either one pole or the other, but not both. We cannot suggest with confidence that the same dimensions would emerge from another sample with other passages. However, the *nature* of the dimensions support the thesis that left and right brain processes are relevant to the ways people organize belief.

Pierce also asked whether men and women used these dimensions differently. The statistical answer was "No:" being male or female, in and of itself, showed no relation to the dimensions. But, in certain instances differences did appear. It is to those differences I direct your attention.

Polar and Nonpolar Realities

Students were classified as liberal, moderate, or conservative, depending upon their view of the authority of Scripture. Liberal women used the dimension of INSTRUMENTAL versus RELATIONAL significantly *less* than other students. Liberal men used the dimension of HUMAN EFFORTS versus DIVINE POWER significantly *more* than other students. Further, liberal women used this third dimension of HUMAN EFFORTS/DIVINE POWER *less* than the other groups of either sex.

These preferences are suggestive. Women reporting a moderate or conservative theology organized belief much the same as men. We inferred that those women had been socialized in the dominant male-oriented culture. In contrast, women who espoused a liberal theology did not organize belief the same as men. They seemed to have resisted conventional socialization.

By the "same as men," I mean a polar dialectic in which instrumental activity and relational activity are opposites and human effort contrasts with divine power. The study was not designed to identify nonpolar cognition, so we cannot say specifically *how* liberal women organize reality. None the less, the data give credence to feminist criticisms of a masculinized science (Bordo [1986] 1987; Rosel [1983] 1987; Harding and O'Barr, 1987)-- Pierce's and mine included. The average male organizes reality in terms of dichotomies and dualities. Polar contrasts -- such as human effort or God's acting, a rational doing or a relational being, a redeeming God or a creating God, proclaiming what is right or manifesting what is real -- do *not* reflect the way women naturally know and intuitively believe.

Other investigators are identifying a similar pattern, namely, that men and women use religious symbols in different ways (Bynum, Harrell, and Richman 1986; Bynum 1987). Building upon Ricoeur's conviction that symbols "give rise to thought" in that they precede thought and so are "opaque, oblique, and analogical." Caroline Walker Bynum, Stevan Harrell, and Paula Richman (1986) marshall cross-cultural evidence to demonstrate the different ways in which women and men experience and use symbols. The evidence shows that within any single tradition, when men and women work with that culture's symbols and myths -- "writing in the same genre, and living in the same religious or professional circumstance" -- they exhibit consistent male/female differences:

> Women's symbols and myths tend to build from social and biological experiences; men's symbols and myths tend to invert them. Women's mode of using symbols seems given to the muting of opposition, whether through paradox or through synthesis; men's mode seems characterized by emphasis on opposition, contradiction, inversion, and conversion. Women's myths

and rituals tend to explore a state of being; men's tend to build elaborate and discrete stages between self and others (Bynum 1986, 13).

The presence or absence of polarities, dichotomies, and dualisms seems to be the difference between men and women in their cognitive style and religious use of symbols.

In a study of "Holy Feast and Holy Fast: The Religious Significance of God To Medieval Women," Bynum (1987) shows that men tended "to construe many aspects of reality in terms of either/or." For them, "symbolic dichotomies and reversals were at [the] very heart" of male experience in the late Middle Ages. Not only did they use the male/female dichotomy as "symbol of authority/nurture, spirit/flesh, law/mercy, strong/weak, but in a broader sense [they used the male/female dichotomy] as a way of expressing the contrast between God and soul, divinity and humanity, clergy and laity." For men, the path of spirituality required a reversal of male dominance into a state of female-identification as "a symbol of dependence on God -- both as a way of describing themselves as cared for by God and as a way of underlining their own renunciation of worldly power and prestige" (Bynum 1987, 281-284). Only thus could the contradiction between divinity and humanity be reconciled in the Incarnation: God-become-man. Crisis of identity, conversion from sinful ways, reversal of role dominance, and the need to embrace the contradictions embedded in opposition and otherness characterized male experience.

Women, in contrast, were not on a hierarchical ladder of roles and statuses as men were. Their perception of reality was one of "continuity" with their social and biological realities (Bynum 1987, 288-294). In their quest for God they became what they already symbolized, namely, "the fleshy, the nurturing, the suffering, the human." Instead of inverting what they were, they deepened their perception of what they were. Their symbols disclosed less contradiction and more "synthesis and paradox."

Quite clearly, women's basic images referred to themselves as "female to a male God or as androgynous." In their symbolizing the "humanity of Christ," they gave the concept of "human" a meaning beyond any dichotomy between male and female. Because of the continuity in the development of themselves, a concept of "other" played little part. They drew on and amplified symbolic aspects of life closer to their ordinary experience, such as eating, suffering, and lactating.

Their sense of self was shaped by the symbolic dichotomies of the dominant theological tradition of proclamation, redemption, and world-transformation. That is true. It is equally true that they appropriated that symbolic cosmos in a different way from men and with different implications for both sexes. Their sense of self was confirmed by continuity with the nondominant theological tradition of manifestation, creation, and world-affirmation.

> It was from age-old notions that God, mind, and power are male whereas soul, flesh, and weakness are female that women drew inspiration for a spirituality in which their own suffering humanity had cosmic significance (Bynum 1987, 294).

Because men were high and lifted up, they needed to be brought low. They had "to renounce their dominance." Women expressed little interest in male/female contrasts. Instead, they deepened their ordinary experience "when God impinged upon it." Their bodies not only served as "a symbol of the humanness of both genders but also a symbol of -- and a means of approach to -- the humanity of God" (Bynum 1987, 295-296). Medieval spirituality presents a contrast between the opposition and otherness in the way men used symbols and the continuity and ordinariness in the way women used symbols.

I speculate that the different ways the brain is organized lead to women perceiving a pattern of cooperation in life and men perceiving a pattern of competition in the universe.

Structural anthropologists have identified ways in which dichotomous symbols tend to reflect and reinforce the power of those who are identified with normative "culture" (Bynum 1987, 293). This is especially true with the basic dichotomy of culture and nature, and by inference, of men and women. Pierce's data (1986) showed that the conventionalized women -- those who took a moderate to conservative view of the authority of Scripture -- used the same polar dimensionality as men in processing both imagistic and analytic information, whereas the theologically liberal women did not. Bynum's research (1987; Bynum, Harrell, and Richman 1986) goes further. It shows that when women voice their spiritual experience, they do so in terms of the continuity of their ordinary life and not in the dichotomies and reversals of male experience (Glaz 1987). This pattern between the sexes has been demonstrated in psychosocial development (Gilligan [1982] 1983; Chodorow [1978] 1979) as well as in philosophy (Harding and Hintikka 1983).

I submit that polarities and dichotomies, characteristic of the dominant (male) culture, arise from the sharp division of labor between left and right brains. That asymmetry is more prevalent among men and, specifically, late maturers in relation to language. The corollary is this: more evenly distributed (bilateral) processes of what is sequential and what is simultaneous, weak asymmetry in technical language, is more prevalent among women and, specifically, early maturers in relation to language. The result of that cognition is a sense of continuity within life experience, identification with others, a participation in the ordinariness of the every day. Incidentally, left handed males are more likely to exhibit processing similar to females than do strongly dominant right handed males.

When avoiding dichotomies, men have tended to view life dialectically. Neither "this" nor "that;" but "this," then "that," for the sake of some yet to be known synthesis. Women, however, reveal a less dialectic process, more "an acceptance of, a continous living with, paradox." Their understanding of God tends to be a process of "reconciliation and continuity." The relationship between "social facts and symbolic meanings" is complex (Bynum, 1986, 14), yet the fact or phenomenon continues: women draw on modes of symbolic discourse different from those of men. Even when the sexes use the same symbols and rituals, these are invested "with different meanings and different ways of meaning." Despite the altar at Chartres, for women food was crucial (Bynum, 1987). An awareness of gender difference enriches "our understanding of both symbol and humanity" (Bynum 1986, 16).

Another Reality

Feminists -- whether from a secular philosophical-political perspective or from a religious-liberation perspective -- dismantle conventional ways of knowing and conventional convictions as to what constitutes truth. These are issues of epistemology, ontology, and theology. The task is twofold, though the process is not necessarily sequential. In technical language, the task is called "deconstruction" on the one hand and "reconstruction" on the other. In biblical imagery, it is Jeremiah hearing the Lord touching his mouth and saying to him:

> Behold, I have put my words in your mouth.
> See, I have set you this day over nations and
> over kingdoms.
>
> *to pluck up and to break down,*
> *to destroy and to overthrow,*
> *to build and to plant*
> (Jeremiah 1:9-10 RSV emphasis added).

The dismantling, deconstructing, plucking up and breaking down calls into question a dichotomized view of reality and/or God. I have alluded to some of the dichotomies. Let me quickly note others: plenitude versus scarcity, value-free versus value-laden, fixed features versus contextual variables, the adversarial method of inquiry versus the affiliative method of inquiry, reason versus emotion, sin versus salvation, objectivity versus subjectivity. The list is endless because our capacity -- and by "our" I mean primarily male capacity -- to dissect, divide, and isolate seemingly is limitless.

"We" (meaning men mostly) continue to argue about whether the sun is more important than the moon. In a rhetorical question I ask: is polarity something which exists in reality? The answer, of course, is "No! Polarities exist in our mind -- especially the left hemisphere -- as we observe, analyze, and seek to control reality."

Further, "we" (meaning men mostly) continue to ignore donkeys. In a rhetorical question I ask: are the minds of men and women the same? The answer, of course, is "No! The average man divides up reality, while the average woman holds reality together."

The reconnecting, reconstructing, planting and building points to the basic integrity of Reality. To make that task explicit philosopher Jane Flax (1985, 269-271) offers ten theses as "the beginning of a feminist theory of knowledge;"

(1) Knowledge has served "a defensive function," stemming as it has from "an arrested" development in childhood which has lacked "true reciprocity."

(2) The seemingly unreconcilable dualisms, to which I have referred, reflect the failure to take into account the earliest period of development "in which the self emerges within the context of a relation."

(3) "The relation between content and method" has failed to include "the 'female' dimensions of experience."

(4) By itself, women's experience is "not . . . an adequate ground for theory. As the other pole of the dualities it must be incorporated and *transcended*" (italics added).

(5) Beyond the "critique of domination," "a new stage of human development is required in which reciprocity can emerge for the first time as the basis of social relations."

(6) Every form of knowledge needs to be reformulated by being "traced back to the life histories and purposes. . . of those who produce it."

(7) Every concept "must be relational and contextual," which means taking into account "the multiplicity of experience, the many layers of any instant in time and space."

(8) Dialectics requires actively thinking "in terms of process, history and interrelationships."

(9) *Experience* needs to be filtered and shaped in "self-reflective and self-critical" ways, that is, it is "not organized on a principle of domination (of race, class, gender, and/or expertise in light of institutional necessity)."

(10) In re-evaluating knowledge and experience, the claim "of objectivity or neutrality" is no more "privileged" than other claims.

Flax identifies an ironic paradox in feminism: namely, that women's desire for liberation requires them to "take on" the philosophical task of identifying Reality -- how we know it, how we know that we know it, and what it is that we know. Historically, women have been identified with bearing children and nurturing life. "Yet precisely because knowing and being cannot be separated," she concludes, "we must know how to be." And that "knowing how to be" means Reality is relational and contextual, not separated and abstract.

Polarity and Domination

In MEDICINE, MIND, AND THE DOUBLE BRAIN, Anne Harrington (1987), an Alexander von Humboldt research fellow in West Germany, clearly demonstrates how brain science, instead of being objective, has reflected "individual, cultural and philosophical prejudices." At their worst, she ties those biases to "an ideology of white male supremacy."

In 1861, physican Paul Broca provided the first scientific evidence that language was located in the left hemisphere. As the "talking" hemisphere, it was called the "major" or the "dominant" hemisphere. Because the right hemisphere was "silent," it was regarded as "minor" or "nondominant" and thereby of lesser value.

While polar pairings -- such as left and right, light and dark, male and female -- have been argued as balanced -- that is, each requires the other in a dialectical process -- in actual fact "they always operate as covert hierarchies; we have trouble imagining difference without domination and subordination. Thus from the very beginning of research on the differences of hemispheric function in the double brain, scientists were attracted to the hypothesis that one hemisphere, the left, must be dominant," and men were more left brained than women, which made their half of humanity the "norm against which all deviants (including women) might be measured." In short, the dual oppositional system of the double brain has "enshrin[ed] certain moral and social discriminations" (Showalter 1987).

I have laid out evidence suggesting that male brains tend to exhibit strong specialization of function. That lateralization makes for an extreme division of labor between the left and right hemispheres, with the result that Reality -- and approaches to Reality -- invariably are dualistic and covertly hierarchical. In addition, female brains tend to exhibit generalization of function. Bilaterality makes for a more distributed process involving both hemispheres, with the result that Reality -- and approaches to Reality -- are invariably relational, contextual, and egalitarian.

The Integrity of Reality and Monotheizing

I now connect my analysis of genes and gender to an understanding of God.

Biblical scholar James A. Sanders (1987b) addressed the phenomenon of fundamentalism in religion and politics by a close analysis of Moses confronting Pharoah and God supposedly "hardening Pharoah's heart" (Exodus 4:21, et al). I say "supposedly" because Sanders found that the Hebrew word translated "hardened" is the same word which, when used in connection with Israel's life, is translated "encouraged."

Nine of the seventeen times the word is used it means "encourage," suggesting that "hardened" may be a misreading. Or, in terms of cognitive processing, to translate the word as "hardened" reflects a dualistic mind-set, one that sees reality and, therefore, perceives God as separate and over against the world. We, especially men, transform a unifying, relational, contextual process into an oppositional, rationalized, set of abstractions. Which is more important -- the sun or the moon, the Israelites or the Egyptians, the Russians or the Americans, women or men?

Sanders insists that the biblical witness is relational, not oppositional. He calls that relational reality "monotheizing" or "the Integrity of Reality." God works in Pharoah exactly as God works in Moses. God works in death just as God works in life. There is no division -- in Reality or in God. Our religious heritage is not polytheistic -- God versus humanity, us versus others, life versus death. Many believers have conceived it so. Faithfulness to tradition, however, requires that we live a monotheizing life, one in which being and knowing are expressions of One Reality, a reality with Integrity.

The feminist criticism voices what the history of patriarchy has muffled, namely, a relational reality of continuity, cooperation, and caring. The monotheizing challenge recalls us to the Integrity of Reality -- a relational reality, a seamless robe which comes from and covers everyone and everything. Research supports the fact that the brains of men and women are organized differently. And that difference makes a difference!

Reconstruction in theology, as in epistemology, directs us toward that more basic bilateralized experience of reality. Theologian Sallie McFague, for instance, in developing *Models of God: Theology for an Ecological, Nuclear Age* (1987), lifts up the relationship between God and the world in a way that goes beyond proclamation and manifestation. Perhaps it is more accurate to say that she recovers a nonpolarized experience of creation and redemption. She does this by experimenting "with the models of God as mother, lover, and friend of the world, and with the image of the world as God's body" (McFague 1987, xi).

In terms of dualism, feminist theologian Rosemary Radford Ruether points out that "[t]he extension and deepening of psychic integration lead women necessarily toward a critique not just of male psychic dualism but also of male sociological dualism. Psychic integration demands a social revolution . . . the crossing of the psychic-social boundaries of the male dualistic world . . . a transformation of the relationship between the spheres of psychic capacities and social roles" (Ruether 1983, 113). According to her and others (Glennon 1979, 97-115):

> Women, building upon psychic integration, seek a new sociological integration that overcomes the schizophrenia of mind and of society. Women want to integrate the public and the private, the political and the domestic spheres in a new relationship that allows the thinking-relational self to operate throughout human life as one integrated self, rather than fragmenting the psyche across a series of different social roles. Women want to tear down the walls that separate the self and society into "male" and "female" spheres. This demands not just a new integrated self but a new integrated social order (Ruether 1983, 113).

My point is made -- the sublety of the obvious can be named: the Godlike takes into account, as necessary for adequate knowing, the experiences of both women and men.

The Godlike knows that men and women differ.

The Godlike knows that no individual bears "the image and likeness of God;" only the species does (Genesis 1:26-27).

The Godlike knows that in Christ Jesus "there are no more distinctions" . . . for we are all one (Galatians 3:28)!

The Godlike knows that the mind of God (to use the title of a recent book on gender [Benderly 1987]) makes a "myth of two minds!"

CHAPTER THREE

COGNITIVE STYLES IN A DOUBLE MIND

If any of you lacks wisdom,
let him [or her] ask God,
who gives to all generously . . .
But let [one] ask in faith,
with no doubting,
for [one] who doubts is like
a wave of the sea that is driven and tossed . . .
a double-minded [person] . . .
will [not] receive anything from the Lord
(James 1:5-8 RSV).

Sixteen year old Paul looked at a single point on a blank screen directly in front of him (Gazzaniga and LeDoux 1978, 146-150, 155; Gazzaniga 1985, 65-73, 88-91). His task was to identify what the researchers flashed to either side of the fixation point. Because of the speed of the exposure, only the hemisphere to which the stimulus was directed would see what was on the screen. The results of the procedure would contribute to what was being learned about the ways the neocortex -- the new brain -- the latest development in the evolution of the brain -- worked.

To the left of the fixation point the researchers flashed a snow scene picturing a snowman, a car covered with snow, and smoke coming from the chimney of a house blanketed in snow. To the right of the fixation point they flashed a chicken claw. Because the left side of the body is controlled by the right hemisphere and the right side of the body is controlled by the left hemisphere, Paul's right hemisphere saw a snow scene while his left hemisphere saw a chicken claw (Figure 6).

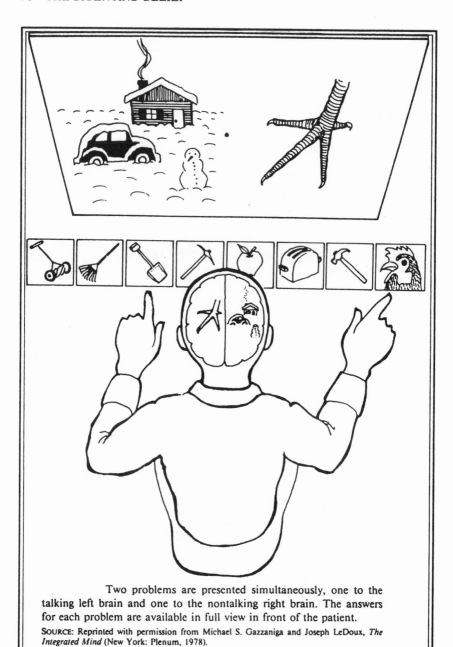

Two problems are presented simultaneously, one to the talking left brain and one to the nontalking right brain. The answers for each problem are available in full view in front of the patient.

SOURCE: Reprinted with permission from Michael S. Gazzaniga and Joseph LeDoux, *The Integrated Mind* (New York: Plenum, 1978).

FIGURE 6. Two different cognitive tasks.

On the table the researchers had spread out eight cards with different objects on each one: a lawnmower, a rake, a shovel, an axe, an apple, a toaster, a hammer, and a chicken head. They asked him to point to the card that went with what he had seen on the screen. In typical split brain fashion his right hand, directed by his left hemisphere, selected the chicken head because it went with the claw; and his left hand, directed by his right hemisphere, picked the shovel because it was associated with the snow scene. Like every patient who had the fiber track cut which carries information from one hemisphere to the other, neither hemisphere knew what the other hemisphere had seen. Each half made different associations while oblivious of the fact that each was seeing a different scene. The halves could not communicate with each other.

Paul was asked, "Why did you do that?" meaning why did he pick the different pictures. He looked at the doctor and replied without hesitating, "Oh, that's easy. The chicken claw goes with the chicken head and you need a shovel to clean out the chicken shed."

How did that explanation come about?

The Hemisphere That Talks

Since 1861, scientists have known that the ability to speak is located in the left hemisphere of most people (Springer and Deutsch [1981] 1985, 9-11; Kolb and Whishaw [1980] 1985, 310-313). In April of that year, physican Paul Broca heard a paper at the Anthropological Society of Paris which claimed that right side paralysis and loss of speech (or aphasia) were the result of damage in the left hemisphere. Broca had a patient named "Tan" who suffered from those deficits. He was called Tan because "Tan" was the only word he uttered.

"Tan" died two weeks later which enabled Broca to perform a post-mortem examination of Tan's brain. The left frontal area was indeed damaged. Broca reported the evidence to the next meeting of the society, though the group received the news with indifference. Ironically, a second autopsy report a few months later was greeted with great excitement. During the next two years he found the same pattern in eight other patients. While he drew no conclusions, the area has been known as Broca's area ever since. Language was assumed to be localized in the left frontal lobe of the neocortex.

Evidence about the localization of language in the left hemisphere led scientists to distinguish between the talking left half and the silent right half. The lack of expressive speech in the right hemisphere led scientists to label it the "minor" or nondominant hemisphere. In contrast, they regarded the left hemisphere as the "major" or dominant hemisphere because it communicated (see Harrington 1987). The right half has continued to be regarded as the silent brain.

Consequently, to ask a patient to say what he or she sees or to explain what he or she has done is to communicate with the patient's left hemisphere, the talking brain. The right brain receives different information without being able to initiate verbal responses about that information. It can point with the left hand but it has no capacity to say what it knows.

There are notable qualifications modifying this generalization. Women and left-handed men present a less distinct pattern of left hemisphere dominance for language (Kolb and Whishaw [1980] 1985, 513-545, 357-369; Springer and Deutsch [1981] 1985, 117-142, 175-185). Researchers Norman Geschwind and Albert Galaburda have estimated that difficulties in the development of a left brain dominance for language may be present in as much as 30 to 35% of the population (Geschwind and Galaburda 1985, 432, 437, 446-447). That fact alone suggests why no one is able to tie up reality into a neat package which applies to everything and everyone. At best we can identify central tendencies and significant variations. Definitive conclusions elude us. We live in an open reality, a reality characterized by patches of recognition and stretches of novelty. Nevertheless, the fact remains that for the great majority of people, language is located basically in the left hemisphere.

For split brain patient Paul to report that he picked the chicken head to go with the chicken claw, therefore, only replicated well-established evidence. What proved unexpected was how his talking left brain handled the information locked in his silent right brain. Remember, the left hemisphere had no way of knowing about the snow scene which the right hemisphere had seen. Yet the left hemisphere did observe that the left hand selected the shovel. Although ignorant of the snow scene, the left hemisphere did know about the shovel. When asked to explain why he had chosen a chicken head with his right hand and a shovel with his left hand, Paul began with the claw/head connection and immediately included the shovel (minus the snow scene) in the explanation.

What happened in Paul's brain?

Left Brain Explanation

His left brain easily explained why it had picked the head after seeing the claw. That half had seen the claw and that half picked the head. In addition, that half had seen the left hand pick the shovel, so it included the shovel in the explanation. Because the talking brain had no internal awareness of the snow scene, it simply guessed at why the left hand had picked the shovel. In other words, it incorporated the mysteriously selected shovel into a supposedly reasonable statement. Of course one would use "a shovel to clean out the chicken shed."

To anyone unaware of the snow scene, Paul's explanation made sense. Only it was a guess, a rationalization, an imaginative construction of why the external world included a claw, a chicken head, and a shovel. The left brain explained the unexplainable in terms of something it regarded as reasonable.

Evidence such as this suggests that the dominant hemisphere for language, usually the left hemisphere, appears to be the source of our explanations as to why things are the way they are. It is "the interpeter" of human experience and physical reality (Gazzaniga 1985; 1988). The left brain constantly is making sense of what it knows and observes. The left brain talks, and what it says is based on what it understands. What it understands appears to be determined as much by what it observes in the outer world as by what it knows directly from the inner world.

Left brain explanation *seems to be objective.* I say "seems to be objective" because data such as Paul's rationalization suggests that knowledge derived from observation may be at odds with knowledge coming from right hemisphere processing. The left hemisphere is the vigilant half of the brain. It notices what goes on; it tags what it sees with verbal labels; it lets us know what is in the public domain. And because it is conscious of its own consciousness, it constructs a rationale which stablizes the world as it perceives the world to be. It is the logical brain.

If the left brain explains everything in a rational way, what of the silent right brain? What does it do?

Right Brain Responsiveness

One neurologist likened the right brain to a traveller in a foreign land. In order to make one's intentions intelligible to the citizens, one has to rely on an interpreter (cited by MacLean 1978, 337). By oneself, the visitor is reduced to frantic gestures and simple words. Nuances of meaning are impossible. Communication consists of a nod of the head and a wave of the hand. The right brain needs the left brain to voice what it knows.

The lack of active speech, however, does not mean that the right brain (or nondominant hemisphere for language) is less important than the left brain (Perecman 1983; Myers 1984; Ardila and Ostrosky-Salis 1984). In fact, increasing evidence supports the centrality of its contribution to language. It gives language the qualities of imagination, pattern-making, and felt-meaning. It is the intuitive brain.

When the right half is impaired, for whatever reason, the person sounds like "a kind of talking computer that decodes [information] literally" (Gardner [1974] 1976, 295-296) without the feeling tone which is present in normal conversation. A person simply is unable to process the symbolic or metaphoric dimension of what is spoken (Heilman, Watson, and Bowers 1983). The emotion in what is said no longer exists; only formal prose remains (Sacks [1970, 1981, 1983, 1984, 1985] 1987, 80-84).

Despite its designation as "minor," there is nothing "minor" about right brain activity (Harrington 1987). Without it we become talking machines -- without emphases, without stories, without genuinely human discourse.

Two Minds

Paul's reaction to two different visual stimuli orients us to differences between the dominant and nondominant hemispheres. St. Paul's struggle between willing one thing and doing another (Romans 7:15-25) and experiences of alternating phases of being Jekyll-like and Hyde-like begin to make sense. Split brain research has led the way to discovering such differences (Springer and Deutsch [1981] 1985, 25-65; Gazzaniga 1970; Sperry 1982). The two hemispheres make up what is known as the neocortex -- that part of the brain which is the latest to develop in the long course of evolution. In order to understand the implications of the new brain for the way our mind works and then for patterns of belief I need to present more about split brain research itself.

Because of difficulty in alleviating the effects of epileptic seizures, during the 1960s a number of patients underwent a radical operation. It involved cutting the fibers which connected their left and right hemispheres. Seizures have been likened to electrical thunderstorms. They originate in one side of the brain, usually the right temporal area, and spread to the other side of the brain as the person becomes totally incapacitated. The separation of the two hemispheres, however, prevented the thunderstorms from causing devastating effects in the sufferer.

By cutting that structure, which is known as the corpus callosum, neither hemisphere had access to the other hemisphere. Neither information nor electrical discharge could be exchanged. All lines of communication were gone. Each half now functioned as an independent mind. Each possessed its own source of information. Each operated according to its own perception of the world. Each reacted according to its own evaluation of what it knew (Sperry 1968). The brain became two minds in one head.

Most of our nervous system crosses from one side to the other (Kolb and Whishaw [1980] 1985, 26-68). That results in the right side of the body being controlled by the left hemisphere while the left side of the body functions under the control of the right hemisphere. The visual system is no exception. What is seen in the left visual field goes only to the right hemisphere, and what is seen in the right visual field goes only to the left hemisphere. With the fiber track connecting the two hemispheres no longer working, split brain patients were responding to two separate and distinct kinds of information.

Since the successful severing of the corpus callosum, investigators have directed attention to people with intact brains as well as those with impaired brains (Springer and Deutsch [1981] 1985, 67-92). Interest has tended to converge on the two hemispheres. The implicit assumption has been that consciousness -- whether explanatory as in the left half or responsive as in the right half -- mirrors reality. It is exactly here that we come upon the connection between the new brain and what I am calling the "old" mind.

The neocortex -- the new brain with its two minds -- gives us clues to understanding the rationality of what I am calling the "old" mind. The talking left hemisphere has been taken mistakenly as the whole mind, or at least the most important part of the brain, the major hemisphere, the essence of the human mind (Harrington 1987).

Making Sense of The Double Mind

As a way to experience the two modes of consciousness of the double brain, I invite you to try a few exercises in perception and sensation.

First, take a blank piece of paper, a pencil or pen, and make a list with numbers 1 to 12 (Zdenek 1983, 129-130). Next, think of twelve words which describe how you think about yourself. This will take a few minutes to do. Once you have finished your list, put it aside. We will come back to it later in the Chapter.

Second, fold your hands. . . . Now fold them the other way. Some people find that request puzzling because they can conceive of no other way to fold them than they actually do. Specifically, if your right thumb and index finger were on top of your left thumb and index finger, reverse them; or if your left thumb and index finger were on top of your right thumb and index finger, reverse that. . . . Now fold your hands the way you usually do.

Were you aware there was another way to fold your hands? Ask people you know to fold their hands. How many do it like you do and how many fold them the other way?

I suggest -- semi-facetiously -- that people go to war over the question of "which is the right way to fold one's hands?" This experience of difference is so subtle that most of us never realize the world could be divided into right-over-left or left-over-right or that some fold their hands either way easily and comfortably. We do what comes "naturally" and never think that others might have a different "natural" pattern. The issue is like Nasrudin settling the argument as to which is more important -- the sun or the moon. The distinctions are arbitrary and only make sense when torn out of context and posited as abstract questions.

These exercises are intended to provide you a sensory experience of the two sides of your body and beyond that of the double mind. The hemispheres deal with different information and also deal with information differently. Two modes of consciousness reflect two sides of the brain (Ornstein [1972, 1977] 1986).

Psychologist Robert E. Ornstein suggests an easy way to become aware of the rational and artistic modes of consciousness (Ornstein [1972] 1977, 18-19). He invites us to close our eyes and attempt to become aware of each side of our body separately. The task is to make the subtle obvious by identifying the feelings and sensations associated with each side in responses to specific contrasts:

> which side is more active and which more passive?

> which side is more logical and which more "intuitive?"

> which side is more feminine and which more masculine?

> which side is "lighter" and which "darker?"

These metaphors have their bodily correlates. The average right-handed person will most likely experience the right side of the body as more active, logical, masculine and lighter, while the left side will most likely be felt to be more passive, intuitive, feminine and darker. A few people experience no such distinctions, but most of us do discern differences when we attend to such instructions.

Try a final exercise to experience the different modes of perception. Take a blank sheet of paper (Zdenek 1983, 142-143). Put your pencil or pen in your nondominant hand, the hand with which you normally do not write. Now list numbers from 1 to 12. Next, write 12 words you feel describe who you are. This will take several minutes and you may feel awkward.

When you finish, compare this second list with the first one you made a while ago. In what ways are they alike? In what ways are they different? People report a variety of differences: words in the second list tend to be shorter, more earthy, more emotional;

words in the first list tend to be longer, more conceptual, more abstract. The second list usually reveals our more vulnerable side. Some of that difference may be because I asked you to "think" of words to write with your dominant hand and to write words with your nondominant hand which you "feel" describe you. The more similar the two lists are the more likely it is your two hemispheres have been communicating with each other. The process of psychotherapy or attending to your dreams can contribute to such exchange.

Information for each list came from different sources in your brain. The first list originated in the left hemisphere or the dominant hemisphere for language and conceptual thought. That applies also for most left-handed people, especially those "hookers" who write with their fingers pointed toward their chest or else shift the paper to take account of the awkward position of the pencil or pen (Springer and Deutsch [1981] 1985, 131-134). The second list originated in the right hemisphere or the nondominant hemisphere which specializes in imagery and emotional expressions.

Exercises like the above reflect what we are learning about the brain and differences between the two hemispheres. The public's fascination with this discovery contributes to the intrigue with neuropsychology. For instance, in *Whole-Brain Thinking: Working From Both Sides of the Brain to Achieve Peak Job Performance,* Jacquelyn Wonder and Priscilla Donovan (1984) translate brain research into ordinary life for the sake of more effective living. New books on the contrast, conflict and complementarity of the two sided brain are appearing regularly. At this point you have an idea how making sense and making meaning go together. The body is the bearer of the double mind. With the body we can access the brain, at least experientially. Such experience helps make the empirical evidence understandable.

Double Mind/Divided Belief

Split brain patients like Paul have alerted us to two streams of consciousness -- one analytic and the other holistic. The new brain can be a double mind. Research has shown how the logical hemisphere can dominate the intuitive hemisphere. That domination has led people to think that the way things are explained is the way things are objectively.

The dualistic tradition has reified the experience of those distinguishable streams of consciousness into basic patterns of the way reality is assumed to be. People have elevated these differences into cosmic certainties. The world gets understood in only one way.

We are now beginning to understand the mechanisms and processes of the double mind. Each hemisphere processes different information differently. As the Nasrudin story of the tea house suggests, people argue over whether the sun or the moon is more important, whether a left brain explanation is more basic than a right brain responsiveness. But the fact that our one brain can be of two minds -- and in some instances of many minds -- is an experience familiar to everyone.

The new brain, however, is not the only way to understand the brain. In fact, to restrict our attention to consciousness itself is to tear us out of our evolutionary environment. The two minds of the one brain actually are more surface appearances than deep reality. Right brain impressions and left brain interpretations are extensions of an inner core; they are not independent centers of self-conscious intention.

The neocortex is the latest development in evolution. That makes it neither supreme nor independent. Only a rationalistic bias could believe the two minds to be absolutes. We are learning from the neurosciences, from the cognitive sciences, and, yes, from theology that conscious cognition eludes our mastery. We are connected to the universe as a whole. It is to that more evolutionary and cosmic connection we turn in understanding the brain as a locus of knowledge in understanding belief.

CHAPTER FOUR

THE TRIUNE BRAIN

EMERGING EVOLUTION

It was you [O God] who created my inmost self,
and put me together in my mother's womb;
for all these mysteries I thank you:
for the wonder of myself,
for the wonder of your works.
(Psalm 139:13-14 JB)

We all have one head (with two cognitive styles) (Restak 1979; Luria 1973; Springer and Deutsch [1981] 1985, 275-283; Geschwind and Galaburda 1984; Benson and Zaidel 1985; Levy 1980a; 1980b; 1985b; Bradshaw and Nettleton 1983). We process sensory input in back of the head and activate motor output in front. The brain includes three levels of complexity (MacLean 1970; 1978), which complexity raises a question about putting too much importance on the double mind of the two hemispheres alone. All complex activity needs the whole brain. Every part must play its part.

Although split brain research has revealed two minds, further inquiry places the analytic and integrative processes in a wider perspective. There is more to consciousness than consciousness itself. We have known that fact because of religious traditions and mystical experiences. We have explored that fact since Freud expounded his view of the dynamic unconscious, what he called primary process in contrast to the secondary process of conscious elaboration. But only recently have the insights of dynamic psychiatry and the evidence of empirical brain science begun to converge (Harris 1986; Winson [1985] 1986; Gardner 1985).

To focus on the two hemispheres apart from the rest of the brain creates a view of the human brain which distorts the meaning-making mammals that we are. A fuller view is required, especially as I connect the ways the brain works with the ways people believe God works.

Undoubtedly you have seen pictures of the brain. However you are not likely to have had the privilege, as I did in the neuroscience course in The Medical School of The University of Rochester, of holding a human brain in your hands, and then learning about its parts by dissecting it. Nor are you likely to have had the privilege, as I had at the invitation of neurosurgeon Douglas Anderson, of being in an operating room for hours as he painstakingly worked to remove a blood clot located deep within the recesses of a patient's right hemisphere.

For these reasons you may not have a vivid three dimensional sense of how the brain is structured. So let me provide you with a quick and ready model of the brain as suggested by neurophysiologist Paul D. MacLean (MacLean 1978) of The National Institute of Health in Bethesda, Maryland. Let me put a brain in your hands.

A Brain in Your Hands

To start from the inside of the brain and work outward, make a fist of one of your hands while keeping your thumb outside. You may prefer to do this with your dominant hand, the hand with which you prefer to write or throw a ball. Your fist ought to look like a reptile, especially a snake lifting its head to survey the territory if you move your hand back and forth. This reptilian-like structure is the oldest section of the brain. Your wrist and forearm correspond to the lower brain stem and spinal cord, though in comparison to the actual size of the reptilian brain represented by your fist they are much smaller.

Next, cup your other hand over the snake-like fist. It should fit like a claw around that oldest part of the brain. MacLean called this second and middle region the limbic system (MacLean 1952), after the Latin word *limbus*, which means "border" and refers to the structures bordering the fluid-filled cavity in the center of the brain.

If you make a fist of each hand and hold them together with your finger nails touching and your thumbs pointing toward you, the area formed by your knuckles and palms corresponds to the limbic region. This is the mammalian brain -- or old cortex -- since we share its features with other mammals as we all evolved from our reptilian ancestors. The area represented by the alignment of your fingernails is the corpus callosum, that giant fiber track which allows each hemisphere to let the other know what it knows.

With the old cortex represented by your fists in front of you, imagine you are wearing a pair of gray winter ski gloves. Now you can see and sense something of the size of the human brain. The gloves correspond to the "bark" of outer gray matter known as the cerebral cortex -- the new cortex or neocortex (as each of these phrases is used interchangeably). Your thumbs facing towards you represent the front of the brain, which includes the most recently evolved prefrontal cortex associated with imagination, anticipation, planning, empathy, and a compassionate identification with the feelings, needs, and suffering of other living things (MacLean 1978, 339-341).

Just a few more identification points before I explain what these structures and areas do.

With your fists-fingernails-gloves still in front of you, the visual cortex is located in the area overlying your little fingers. The auditory cortex would be on the back of your hands just below your middle knuckles. Your middle fingers correspond to the motor cortex. By wiggling those middle fingers you have an idea of the area which generates voluntary movements. The mouth and face lie closest to the middle knuckle; the leg and foot are located near the first joint; the rest of the body comes in between (see Hooper & Teresi [1986] 1987, 40). Similarly, your ring fingers and knuckles correspond to the sensory cortex.

Unlike the bony structure of your hands, however, the brain itself, as MacLean puts it, "feels much like a ripe avocado." Facts may or may not be hard, but they are the result of "a soft brain" (Hooper & Teresu [1986] 1987, 45-46).

Brain activity involves a yes/no-go pattern of neuronal excitation-inhibition which results in integrated action. However, the nervous system is now believed to work by a combination of the digital or binary ("yes-no" or "all-or-none") principle with an analogue ("how much") principle (Kolb and Whishaw [1980] 1985, 49). The analogue function of the dendrites (so called because of the Greek word meaning tree), which branch out from every nerve cell, integrates many sources of information. The digital activity, which resides in the single axon (from the Greek word meaning axle), passes on a summary of the input received by the cell to other cells (Kolb and Whishaw [1980] 1985, 32). Everything we do results from our combining discrete processes of either "yes-go" or "no-stop" with continous and graded processes of "a little more" and "a little less."

One further piece of information provides background for my use of the brain in understanding beliefs. In terms of our limited lay knowledge at least, the source of initiative, that locus or origin from which activity springs, resides within both our brain and environment (Gardner 1985; Livingston 1978). Brain and environment interact. No brain without an environment and no environment without a brain -- such is the nature of living reality.

Now that you have an idea of a brain in your hands I describe the brain in more detail. But where to start? There is no one way to describe it.

I could say more about our higher functions as these are generated by the gray matter of the neocortex. Or, I could approach it in terms of the physiological organization of the nervous system with its neuronal structure, electrical activity within the nerve cells and the neurotransmitter activity between nerve cells (Kolb and Whishaw [1980] 1985, 31-61). Or again, I could describe it in terms of its three working systems (Luria 1973, 43-101): the altering system which regulates tone and arousal, the receiving system which takes in and stores information, and the using system which programs activity by organizing consciousness.

Instead, I start with the old brain and not the new brain, with the perspective of evolution (Kolb and Whishaw [1980] 1985, 80-86; Jerison 1985) and not the research on split brains. I take the view which connects us with other mammals and with reptiles and thereby with the physical universe.

MacLean articulates a similar conviction. "Starting with the subjective self as its province (its territory)," he writes, "the domain of evolutionary psychiatry encompasses both the microscopic and macroscopic aspects of all the underlying phenomena as they seem to unfold in past-present-future and *relate to the cosmos*" (MacLean 1985b, italics added). With his concept of The Triune Brain, "a mind of three minds" (MacLean 1970; 1978), he makes that developmental perspective intelligible. MacLean identifies three levels of organization in the brain as a whole (Figure 7).

Levels of Organization

We possess three minds, not two. Each mind reflects three levels of complexity and three stages in evolution. Each mind has its own intelligence, its own data, its own sense of space and time, and its own memory bank. If we do not press the analogy too far, the levels may be associated with a linear view of time: level one locates us in the past, level two relates us to the present, and level three directs us toward the future.

Level One is the oldest region, the Reptilian-like Brain or what MacLean calls The Primal Mind. Here we find the basic instincts and ritual behaviors of precedent. In human terms we might say that this Primal Mind deals with "our territory," "our literal place" in the world. Instinctual behaviors include the "prosematic" non-verbal communication of reptiles, their display behaviors which signal to others who they are, where they are, and what they want: signature, challenge, courtship, and interaction with other creatures, including submissive behavior. These behaviors on our part signal to others who we are and what we are about. The primal mind is territorial -- my place, my prerogative, my space, my inherited niche in the scheme of things. Remember your one fist as a snake's head surveying its environment.

Level Two is the midregion, the Old Mammalian Brain -- the old brain -- or what MacLean calls The Emotional Mind. Here we find a shift from the display behavior of our reptilian connection to the symbolic communication of our mammalian connection. This region generates emotion which gives us "a sense of [the] reality of [ourselves] and the environment and a conviction of what is true and important" (MacLean 1970, 347). In effect, if the reptilian level deals with our physical "place," at this level we are motivated to maintain and enhance our psychological "place." Here is the center of activity necessary for survival, the preservation of the self and the continuity of the species, the Four F's" of the neurobiological joke: feeding, fighting, fleeing, and sexual activity (Hooper and Teresi [1986] 1987, 43).

Recall that your fists with your fingernails touching suggests the way this area appears. The actual structures, however, are claw-like as they cup themselves over the top of the brain stem. (You will find a picture of the limbic region in Figure 8.) The mammalian brain is crossed so that, with the exception of the sense of smell, most incoming information and most outgoing commands

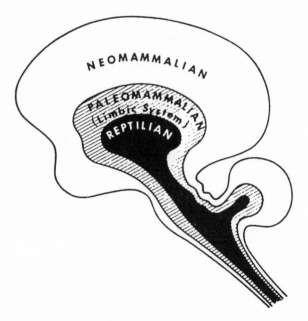

The primate forebrain. In evolution, the primate forebrain expands in hierarchic fashion along the lines of three basic patterns that may be characterized as reptilian, paleomammalian, and neomammalian (from MacLean, 1967).

FIGURE 7. Primate forebrain in evolution.

travel from the left side of the body to the right hemisphere and back to the left side and from the right side of the body to the left hemisphere and back to the right side (Kolb and Whishaw [1980] 1985, 26-28).

As I have indicated, the limbic system makes up much of this old mammalian level. We are motivated by its three main divisions (MacLean 1970). The amygdalar system -- so named because of the almond-shaped amygdala -- involves "self-preservation as it pertains to behavior involved in feeding and the struggle to obtain food." The septal system -- named after the hedge-like septum -- includes "sociability and the procreation of the species." Finally, at least in terms of my simplified account, the thalamocingulate division generates behavior related to family behavior: nursing involved in maternal care, audiovocal communication in the separation call which serves to maintain contact between mother and offspring, and play (cf. Turner 1983). MacLean proposes that the separation call "may be the most basic mammalian vocalization" (MacLean 1985a). The old brain and family life appear to evolve together (MacLean 1982; cf. Trevarthen 1986).

The evolutionary advance from Neanderthal to Cro-Magnon human beings came with the development of the forehead from low brow to high brow features. That expansion contains the prefrontal cortex, a part intimately linked with the thalamocingulate division, which in our brain-in-the-hands model is represented by the thumbs facing towards us. This cortex, as I have said, is the locus of our anticipating, our planning, our capacity for empathy, and our altruistic sentiments.

In addition to these limbic functions of self-preservation, continuity of the species, and nurturing care of the young we find a further function, namely, memory. Memory is associated, in part, with the hippocampus, so named because of the Greek word and its resemblance to the small, marine sea horse. The process involves incorporating highly organized and emotionally laden information into a sense of the continuity of reality (Winson 1986, 30-34, 201-202).

What is novel and unfamiliar gets our attention. We are aroused, alert to unexpected demands, on guard as though our very survival were at stake. We select information, sort it, filter it, take it in according to whether it is pleasurable or painful, desirable or undesirable, to be approached or to be avoided. Over a period of about three years, the hippocampus helps consolidate that new information from the neocortex with information stored in the long term memory. Without that transformation of sensory input from an immediate present into a stabilized past we have little sense of self and little orientation in time and space. We simply are unable to "remember" who we are, where we are, and what we are about. One then lives in the hell of an eternal present, without the recent past and without a usable furture (Kolb and Whishaw [1980] 1985, 481-494; Winson [1985] 1986, 10-17; Hooper and Teresi 1986, 206).

Level Three, which contains the forebrain or neocortex, MacLean calls the New Brain or The Rational Mind. Here we find activity which we take to be distinctly human, most particularly, that which "promotes the preservation and procreation of ideas" (MacLean 1978, 332). As "[m]other of invention and father of abstract thought" (MacLean 1978, 332), the neocortical region, with its two hemispheres, is the locus necessary for the development of culture. It serves as the place which activates and transmits culturally significant information by interacting with the rest of the brain "to produce the cultural modifications of genetic information that is characteristic of humans" (Burhoe 1987; 1973; see Turner 1983).

The complexity of 100 billion neurons, or nerve cells, with something in the neighborhood of 100 trillion connections between them (Hoffman 1987), makes the brain "the most complicated constellation of behaving entities" we know of in the universe (MacLean 1970, 347). The brain combines quite specific programming with remarkable flexibility. Such a characterization, I propose, describes what people have meant through the centuries when they have spoken of an ever-present (that means remarkable flexibility) and an ever-caring (that involves quite specific programming) God.

For me the human brain provides a vision of how God is God. In understanding the brain's complexity, that sense of awe can change into a felt knowledge of its Creator because no matter how much we learn about ourselves we know we did not create ourselves. We are utterly dependent on "a sovereign system of evolving reality which created [us] and all other things . . . Hence [we] must seek to adapt to the unavoidable requirements for living imposed by that superior system of reality -- or else lose life, cease to be" (Burhoe 1973, 415). Our insistent search for meaning reflects the fact that we are forever looking for the Creator God of the universe.

The New Brain

At first glance, the two halves of the brain, like a brain-in-the-hands model, appear to be the same. But just as our hands are different, so too the hemispheres are different, both in their structures and functions (Bryden 1982; Bryden and Ley 1983; Kolb and Whishaw [1980] 1985, 326-356). In effect, our one brain is a double brain (Dimond 1972; Levy 1985a; Bradshaw and Nettleton 1983 (Table 2).

Although evidence is accumulating that some preferential hemisphere patterns are present (Springer and Deutsch [1981] 1985, 205-216), by and large, in lower animals each half performs the same functions (see Denenberg 1983). In humans, however, we find a division of labor between the two hemispheres. Each half specializes -- the left in analytic processing and the right in integrative processing. The way these processes shift to one side or the other is called "laterality," and the result of laterality is known as cerebral asymmetry. The two brains are not the same by virtue of the fact they perform different tasks (Springer and Deutsch [1981] 1985).

TABLE 2   MAJOR FEATURES OF THE CEREBRAL HEMISPHERES

	Dominant* (Left) Brain	Nondominant* (Right) Brain
GENERAL FEATURES		
oriented to	concepts	impressions
type of thinking	logical	associative
direction of attention	narrow focus	broad focus
interested in	specific & realistic	tangible & symbolic
takes the lead in	rational strategy	relational strategy
SPECIAL FEATURES		
input process based on	item-by-item observation, i.e., detached perspective sequential & serial method temporal analysis abstracts parts categorizes generalizes	all-at-once participation, i.e., personal perspective simultaneous & parallel method spatial synthesis attends to patterns images unifies
output process based on	step-by-step deliberate responses slow controlled convergent a fixed structure of procedures & principles formal language style	leaps of inference varied responses rapid spontaneous divergent a flexible approach of trial-and-error pragmatic informal language style

*In most people the left hemisphere is dominant for language and related conceptual processes and the right hemisphere is not, i.e., is nondominant for these. In a small minority of the population the right hemisphere is dominant for language and so the left hemisphere is nondominant.

The evidence supporting these differences is more relative than absolute (Kolb and Whishaw [1980] 1985, 352; Ashbrook 1984a). Any generalization may be inaccurate as far as it applies to any particular hemisphere or person. Complex activity is "complex" by virtue of its dependence upon input from most, if not all, parts of the brain. Even as we describe central tendencies, we must not ignore significant variations in cerebral asymmetry (Kolb and Whishaw [1980] 1985, 357-381).

The Left Half

The dominant brain for language, usually the left hemisphere, processes information analytically (Gazzaniga 1974, 367-382; Levy-Agresti and Sperry 1968; Levy 1974). It deals with information in an item-by-item and step-by-step manner. This narrow logical style includes only a few items in any one category of information (Kinsbourne 1982). It concentrates on detailing small differences between stimuli. Because of that precision it constructs a view of reality which is strictly rational.

As split brain patient Paul revealed, the talking brain builds an orderly world according to what it observes. Even if the data are misrepresented, the world makes sense in that it can be explained logically. The left brain develops what Michael Gazzaniga and Joseph LeDoux call "an attitudinal view of the world involving beliefs and values" (Gazzaniga and LeDoux 1978, 155). That individual view becomes "a dominant theme." Everything, therefore, is reasonable in its own eyes.

The eagle-eyed vigilance of the left hemisphere sharpens attention. The left half takes the lead from the right in processing everything it perceives as requiring a step-by-step analysis (Levy and Trevarthen 1976; Levy 1982). That assertive stance applies to sensory input and motor output alike (Table 3).

The back or posterior region works in a conceptual way. It distinguishes objects by sharpening differences between them. Then it labels these differences so as to make the objects appear to be dis-

TABLE 3 MAJOR SENSORY SYSTEMS OF THE LEFT BRAIN

General Features:
    Vigilant-Rational   Intention
    ● sharpens differences among stimuli
    ● isolates senses from each other

    Interpretive-Explanatory Mental Scheme
    ● input: digital item-by-item strategy which is
        conceptual
        abstract
    ● output: deductive step-by-step strategy which is
        rational
        specialized

Major Sensory Systems:
    Auditory Hearing (Temporary Lobe)
    ● sounds translated into concepts
    ● speech and writing which are
        ideational
        narrow meaning of words
        prosaic/abstract denotative

    Visual Sight (Occipital Lobe)
    ● observation
    ● perspective, that is
        a fixed position
        realistic
        objective
    ● permanence, that is,
        common sense
        basic elements, which are
            separate
            isolated
            repeatable
    ● fixed visualization

    General Sensory (Parietal Lobe)
    ● tension
    ● deliberate responses, which are
        slow
        controlled
        convergent
        refined sensations
        stable

crete entities. By understanding the world from a fixed position, it assumes the world to be as we perceive it, existing entirely apart from us. Reality is fixed, permanent, objective. And we can know that reality by generalizing inductively from separate parts to a supposed whole.

The front anterior region is intentional. By abstracting formal principles from sensory input and translating those principles into specific actions, it enables us to act deliberately. Information is analyzed in terms of basic assumptions. Conclusions are based on a logic which moves from general principles to specific instances. Because of its ability to abstract, it can miss the immediate context. As with the Nasrudin story of the donkey and its goods, attention to details can blind it to the obvious.

In brief, a left brain approach shapes reality rationally. It observes what goes on in the external world. It organizes those observations in terms of definite categories. Based on that clarity, the hemisphere then explains what it has seen in a reasonable way. The posterior area "labels" and "names" objects; the anterior area "analyzes" and "systematizes" the data. Thus the dominant hemisphere specifies what needs to be taken into account if we are to accomplish what we want. In conventional terms it is "content" oriented.

Some evidence associates the dominant hemisphere with a mood pattern called "tarnishing" (Bear and Fedio 1977; Mandell 1980).[1] When the left brain fails to function normally, people tend to dull, spoil, or taint their perception of reality. They give the impression of being done in by what is happening. They report tottering on the edge of catastrope. They exaggerate their mood into either depression or disaster.

The Right Half

In contrast to the left half, the right hemisphere processes information in a holistic or integrative way (Gazzaniga 1974; Levy 1974; Perecman 1983; Ardila and Ostrosky-Solis 1984). By grouping together "a wide variety of similar objects or concepts . . . paying little attention to detail or differences" (Kinsbourne 1982), it works broadly or all-at-once and by leaps of imagination. Because it emphasizes similarities, it blurs differences, thereby creating a world characterized by a web of associations, or a mosaic of meaning. It integrates the senses into natural patterns of relatedness made up of impressions and imagination.

I suggest this activity reflects what we are learning about "the bodily basis of meaning, imagination, and reason" (Johnson 1987; Lakoff 1987). The right half responds impressionistically to the broad features of the environment. That is meaning-making. It comes at "reality" from inside the context. Meaning results from its being part of the drama (in contrast to someone viewing the scene from the audience or off stage) (Mountcastle 1976, 41).

The right half responds quickly, regarding as its domain whatever cannot be classified. It takes the lead from the left hemisphere in processing such information (Levy and Trevarthen 1976; Levy 1982). That priority in responsiveness includes both sensory input and motor output (Table 4).

The posterior region responds to stimuli impressionistically. The result is kaleidoscopic, stereoscopic, ever-changing, ever-vivid, ever-meaningful. Because it responds from inside a context, everything is experienced emotionally (Kolb and Whishaw [1980] 1985, 546-561), or taken personally, in contrast to the supposedly objective left brain. Objects are associated in terms of how they appear rather than in terms of their functional connection. The right brain would associate an open pair of scissors with a crossed knife-and-fork because they looked alike, while the left brain would associate the scissors with needle-and-thread or a knife-and-fork with a piece of cake (Levy and Trevarthen 1976) because they served the same function. The process generates metaphorical meaning and symbolic significance.

TABLE 4 MAJOR SENSORY SYSTEMS OF THE RIGHT BRAIN

General Features:
Relational-Responsive Intouchness
● minimize differences among stimuli
● combine senses

Expressive-Experiential Mental Images
● input: Inferential all-at-once strategy which is
    perceptual
    concrete (tangible)
● output: analogic/metaphoric imaginative strategy involving
    relational connections
    synthetic/holistic patterns

Major Sensory Systems:
General Sensory (Parietal Lobe)
● relaxation
● natural responses, which are
    rapid
    spontaneous
    divergent
    patterned
    varying

Visual Sight (Occipital Lobe)
● participation
● perception, which means
    a personal vantage point
    symbolic content
    subjective meaning
● impressions, which include
    changing scenes
    changing elements, which are
        distinct
        connected
        unique
● flowing impressions

Auditory Hearing (Temporal Lobe)
● sounds not conceptualized
● speech and writing which are
    vivid
    broad meanings
    metaphoric/imaginative
    connotations

The anterior region intuits feeling tone or emotional meaning. Even though it cannot put what is going on into words, it does grasp the data, for instance, what to do with an object such as a fork (Nathan 1969, 276). Because it reacts rapidly, in contrast to the systematic approach of the left brain, it relies on a trial-and-error approach to problem-solving.

In brief, the right brain processes information in a relational manner. It creates a web of connections by linking every part with every other part. That patterning makes the whole accessible through the parts -- *pars pro toto*, substituting a part for the whole, such as a few notes of a song or a few lines of a caricature or a scent which revives a memory (Watazlawick 1978, 69-73). The posterior area "immerses" us in what is immediately meaningful; the anterior area "expresses" or "imagines" a pattern based on a leap of inference. The "logic" of "what is there" depends upon the felt-meaning of "how things appear to be." It takes the lead in assessing the emotional aspects of situations. In conventional terms it is "context" oriented.

In regard to differences in the emotional views of the world by the two brains, some evidence indicates that the right hemisphere tends to "polish" experience (Bear and Fedio 1977; Mandell 1980). Whether its reaction is one of "indifference" or not, right half responses tend to overestimate good feelings and underestimate negative circumstances.[2]

What Is Brain? What Is Mind? Caution and Clarification

Whether we examine data related to the triune brain and its three levels of organization or data associated with the two hemispheres of the neocortex, the data are open to contrasting, even contradictory, interpretations (Bryden 1982; Wong 1984; Ashbrook 1984c, 57-60, 94-96, 320-324). Much of the evidence is ambiguous (Ashbrook 1984a).

Part of that ambiguity, according to scientist-theologian Ralph Wendell Burhoe (1987), arises because the meaning of the term "brain" may involve subjective experience as well as "an objective system requiring objective rules and evidences of causes and effects." Equally pertinent, the term "mind" may refer to subjective experience as well as "to meaning some entity external to conscious experience . . ." Thus, in analyzing "either subjective experience or the presumed object of such an experience . . . the brain become[s] a new and important [instrument] for understanding the objective source (under such categories as nature, God, and brain) for subjective experience." As Burhoe points out, "objectivity" simply refers to that "category of experience where we have learned [that] many experiences have been associated with a common context" (Burhoe 1987).

"Brain" and "mind" are interchangeable terms and thereby equivalent. As the subjective experience of objects, the brain is mind; as an objective system external to conscious experience, the mind is brain. These are not different, even though we can distinguish between physical or mental or spiritual dimensions. In both its mechanisms and its general experience, as Burhoe (1987) describes it, the brain engages in a "restless search of itself to make better sense and order of what is going on." "Brain" and "mind" are not interchangeable terms to the extent I use the word "brain" to refer specifically to biochemical activity which can be identified with objective instruments such as an electroencephalogram or CT scan and "mind" to refer specifically to experiential patterns which are capable of being consciously discerned and described.

In contrast to a dualism or even a sophisticated interactionism, I assume a radical monism. This emergent view (cf. Sperry 1969; 1977) of higher cortical activity -- the activity of *human* animals -- neither negates biochemical processes by an exclusive attention to the supposedly transcendent nor reduces that vivid personal experience of a sense of self, a self of humor, and a sense of deity at the interface with sensory input (Taylor 1979, 17-19) to the supposedly biochemical. The new brain depends upon and is an extension of the old brain.

Current breakthroughs in psychobiological research are eliminat-
ing the gap between mind and body (Rossi 1986; Skinner 1987;
Harris 1986; Ornstein and Sobel 1987) or mind and brain. The
brain, primarily in the limbic-hypothalamic system of the Emotional Mind, coordinates what we refer to conventionally as "mind-
body communication." The materiality of brain produces the
meaningfulness of mind and the purposefulness of mind exists in
and through and because of the physicality of brain. Call it brain-
mind, if you want. The hyphen says the two words belong to one
reality. From a linguistic point of view, therefore, I am using the
terms "brain" and "mind" interchangeably *and* metaphorically (cf.
Ashbrook 1984c, 15-21). The term "mind" identifies the *human*
meaning of the term "brain," even as the term "brain" designates
the *empirical* referent of the term "mind."

I combine the inside characteristics of brain -- all the visceral, perceptual, imaginative, conceptualized learning of viable responses
(Johnson 1987; Lakoff 1987) -- with the outside sources in our history and the communities which express that heritage (Burhoe
1987). As split patient Paul demonstrated, we explain what we experience and observe in rational ways, ways that make sense to us
at the time. In so doing, we are meaning-making creatures (Kegan
1982), creatures wired to make sense of all the information we
process. In religious language that is known as cosmos-making,
creating order out of chaos. Because of that way of interacting
with the world, we are "believing" organisms (Gazzaniga 1985;
Trevarthen 1986; Ross 1986; Henry 1986), "from [belief in] the
hardness and solidity of the floor to our highest spiritual beliefs
about our ultimate destiny and concerns" (Burhoe 1987).

Our brain is the origin of all *human* activity. It is the source of
every interpretation of what is really real and truly right. That
locus of reality, therefore, constitutes a focus for our comprehend-
ing everything. We can use the brain as a way to understand God's
presence in ourselves and in the world in which we live. In the
words of Santiago Ramon y' Cajal (1852-1934), the acknowledged
"maestro" of the microscopic study of the brain:

As long as the brain is a mystery, the universe, [which is] the reflection of the structure of the brain, will also be a mystery (quoted by Feindel 1975, xxvi).

If we take the myth of Genesis 2:6-7 ("a mist went up from the earth and watered the whole face of the ground. Then the Lord God formed _adam_ from the dust of the ground and breathed in _adam's_ nostrils the breath of life; and _adam_ became a living being" JB) as metaphorical language, then the physical and the human -- brain and mind -- are connected. Divine purpose permeates physical matter, even as physical matter discloses transcendent purposing. By combining Cajal's conviction and the Genesis vision, the reality of our brain reflects the reality of a universe full of meaning.

Summary

In the early research on split brain patients, the left hemisphere was thought to deal with verbal information and the right hemisphere with nonverbal information. Subsequent study revealed that to be simplistic (Springer and Deutsch [1981] 1985, 48-49, 79-81). A more accurate interpretation points to the different styles or strategies each brain uses in problem solving. The focus shifted from "what" information is processed to "how" information is processed.

The specialization, however, probably is "not an all-or-none phenomenon." Rather, it falls on "a continuum" of more one style than the other (Springer and Deutsch [1981] 1985, 64). Table 2 lists the main features of the two hemispheres, while Tables 3 and 4 list the specific features of the major sensory systems -- hearing, seeing, and general sensing -- in terms of either an analysis of "constituent parts" in a left brain style or a synthesis of basic ("primitive") wholes in a right brain style (Bever 1975, 252-254, 260). Even though the tables are arranged in separate categories, remember both the "continuum" nature of the features and the intricate complexity of the data.

The left brain works in a rational-explanatory way; the right discloses a relational-experiential mode. That is why I regard the left half as more vigilant and the right half as more responsive, the left as more analytic and the right as more integrative. Neither, however, acts by itself. Each depends upon what the other contributes. Together they make for a unified consciousness and integrated behavior, even when we are "not ourselves," as St. Paul described in the seventh chapter of Romans.

Although the new brain handles information in two distinguishable ways, the halves are extensions of the emotional mind of the old mammalian brain. These higher functions are outgrowths of that core region. In fact, whether we use an analytic or integrative strategy depends upon decisions we make in the limbic system below the level of consciousness (MacLean 1978; 1983; Wilke 1981, 33-56). The decision is an emotional decision: is the situation an encouraging one, which results in a relaxed cooperation with others, or an endangering one, which triggers the fight/flight syndrome of stress?

Neurosurgeon Wilder Penfield claimed that "the *indispensable substratum* of consciousness lies outside the cerebral cortex, probably in . . . the higher brain stem" (Penfield 1975, 19). This is why the hemispheres are not the "highest level" of integration. They function at the "top" of our head, but are "an elaboration level, divided sharply into areas for distinct functions," such as sensory, motor, and psychical or mental (Penfield 1975, 44-48). Human rationality derives from emotional meaning.

In the limbic system we determine whether what is happening to us is disagreeable and painful or agreeable and pleasant. If painful, it calls for an active sharpening of the boundaries between ourselves and the environment. We experience boundary sharpening as tension. If we perceive what is happening is agreeable, then we loosen the boundaries as we accommodate to the situation. We experience boundary-blurring as relaxation. Tension and pain vs. relaxation and pleasure (Table 5).

TABLE 5 MAJOR FEATURES OF THE LIMBIC SYSTEM:[1]

Limbic derives from the word "limbus," which means "forming a border around." The systems consists of a ring of curved structures appearing to nest inside each other. It is a core processing system, neither directly sensory nor motor, dealing with information taken from events, memories of events, and emotions associated with these events and essential in using experience to guide future activity.

Septum (hedge-like membrane on the front section of each fornix)
    Functions within the Limbic System
    ● relaxation with what is familiar
    ● reality of the environment and sociability
    ● procreation and the continuity of the species
    ● nurture of others, especially the young

    Projection to the Right Hemisphere
    ● holistic/symbolic relationships
    ● accommodative activity
    ● boundary relaxing and boundary blurring, that is
        - parasympathetic system
        - energy conserving
        - trophotropic stability and equilibirum

Amygdala (a brain nucleus or assembly of cells lying in front of each
        hyppocampus)
    Functions within the Limbic System
    ● arousal with what is unfamiliar
    ● reality of the self
    ● preservation of the self
    ● fight-flight reaction

    Projections to the Left Hemisphere
    ● analytic/causal connections
    ● assertive activity
    ● boundary sharpening and boundary building, that is,
        - sympathetic system
        - energy-expending
        - ergotrophic arousal

Hippocampus (an elongated, sausagelike structure inside the inner wall of
        each temporal cortex)
    ● memory-affective processing
    ● assimilate the strange into the familiar
    ● conviction of what is true and important

Thalamocingulate Division
    ● familiar-related behavior
    ● nursing and maternal care
    ● audiovocal communication and the separate cell

---

[1] Adapted from Winson (1985) 1986, 33; MacLean 1970; d'Aquili 1983.

The processes of the autonomic nervous system parallel those at the cerebral level. Psychiatrist Eugene d'Aquili shows this by means of a model of energy-expansion, associated with arousal of the sympathetic nervous system (or the ergotropic system), and of energy-conservation, associated with the parasympathetic nervous system maintaining the stability of our bodily activity (or the trophotropic system) (d'Aquili 1983). The amaydala triggers survival behavior which involves self-preservation, such as feeding and fighting. In activating negative associations to stimuli, or by decreasing positive associations, we use the vigilant strategy of the left hemisphere. In contrast, the septum motivates behavior expressive of sociability and so is related to the preservation of the species, such as preliminaries of sexual activity. In positive associations to stimuli we use the responsive strategy of the right hemisphere.

The "logic" of the limbic system is nonlinear. That means its neural pathways are "always bi-directional." They are capable of both tension and relaxation. Emotional convictions can mobilize support for the opposite side of any issue, as we know only too well when we find ourselves caught in a power struggle with others over what is right in a particular situation. In the limbic response, everything happens at once, "with gradual changes in threshold rather than discrete changes of state" (Wilke 1981, 33).

In other words, the different strategies of the neocortex give evidence of an interactive process between ourselves and the emerging universes of influence of which we are a part. These universes include family, society, and value commitments, or what I am identifying as patterns of belief. Ultimately, our cognitive activity serves optimal evolutionary adaptation by combining information from our inner world with information from our outer world. The result is a new level of evolution, what Burhoe describes as "the symbiosis of cultural and genetic heritages as generated by religions" (Burhoe 1987).

As the fullest expression of cultural-biological activity, religion maintains and enhances our "ecological niche" (Burhoe 1981, 120). In both personal and institutional ways, religion can enlarge the possibility of altruistic cooperation. The Book of Leviticus characterizes the transition from kin relationships, as inscribed in the genetic code, to nonkin relationships, as developed in our cultural codes:

> If a stranger lives with you in your land . . . You must count him as one of your own countrymen and love him as yourself -- for you were once strangers yourselves in Egypt (Leviticus 19:34 JB).

We are instructed to respond to everyone as we would respond to ourselves. As human beings, we are more alike than different. The neocortex constructs strategies to deal with, explain, and evaluate the interaction which fits us and our environment together, but it is the limbic system, MacLean insists, which brings "a sense of concern for the welfare of all living things" (MacLean 1983, 370-371).

Conscious activity, therefore, seeks the best adaptive relationship which is possible at any particular moment. When something is amiss -- problematic, unusual, unintelligible, or threatening -- the delicate balance of the limbic system activates the emergent features of our cognition. Our subcortical regions -- reptilian and mammalian centers -- and our cortical regions -- left and right hemispheres -- combine. The result is what scientist-philosopher Michael Polanyi termed "an active shaping of experience performed in the pursuit of truth" (Polanyi 1966, 6).

In being aware of itself the human brain discloses features that transcend the brain itself. This means that the brain seems to understand its own functioning. By virtue of its efforts to explain its own reflection, the brain transcends itself. To understand the brain it is necessary, therefore, that we come to a new understanding of the mind. The whole brain -- the old brain as much as the new brain -- is involved in knowing who we are and knowing the universe of which we are a part.

NOTES

1. Evidence related to personality and emotional correlates of lateralization and interpretation of the evidence are controversial. Some researchers have argued that hemisphere impairment prevents an inhibition of the other hemisphere's process, while others contend impairment only intensifies the process of that hemisphere (see Tucker 1981; Kolb and Whishaw [1980] 1985, 546-572; Heilman and Satz 1983). Tucker (1981), for instance, claims that the left hemisphere is more associated with positive emotions and the right hemisphere more with negative emotions, in contrast to the data and interpretation upon which I draw. A "more parsimonious" and compelling interpretation identifies the right hemisphere "as being more involved than the left in all aspects of emotional behavior" (Kolb and Whishaw [1980] 1985, 561).

2. Right-handed subjects with characteristically higher right hemisphere (than left hemisphere) arousal showed "an optimistic bias, particularly for the left visual field," while subjects with strong right visual field advantages had "a pessimistic bias for rating performance" (Levy, Heller, Barich, and Burton 1983). In personal conversation, Levy indicated that left hemisphere dominance "leveled or neutralized affect." In contrast, weak right hemisphere dominance was associated with a pessimistic biasing, while strong right hemisphere dominance disclosed an optimistic biasing of interpretation.

CHAPTER FIVE

HOW WE KNOW WHAT WE KNOW

*Now faith is the assurance
of things hoped for,
the conviction of things not seen . . .
By faith we understand that the world
was created by the word of God,
so that what is seen
was made out of things which do not appear.
(Hebrews 11:1,3 RSV)*

We live in a voiceless universe. As such it seems like a mindless reality. Yet we long for the universe to speak to us, to show us its life, to share its secrets, to disclose its mindfulness. We struggle to make sense of its vastness and to cope with its strangeness. From time eternal, humanity has worked to understand this reality, to explain its mechanisms, to influence the course of its destiny. There is no way we cannot *not* make sense of the world. Our mind is the meaning-making organ of the universe!

But the puzzle persists: what is mind and what is brain? is the brain actually mind or is the mind only the brain? how do they differ or, more accurately, how are they *distinguishable* and what difference does that make, especially in light of the fact that we are meaning-making creatures?

In his *Confessions*, Augustine expressed the longing to distinguish between physical reality and psychic meaning. He did that by wondering about what is God and what is not God:

> And what is this God? I asked the earth . . . and everything in the earth . . . the sea and the deeps and the creeping things, and they [all] replied, "We are not your

God; seek above us." . . . I asked the heavens, the sun, moon, and stars; and they answered "Neither are we the God whom you seek." And I replied to all these things which stand against the door of my flesh: "You have told me about my God, that you are not [God]." Tell me something about [God]." And with a loud voice they all cried out, "[God] made us" (Augustine 1955, Bk. X, VI, 206).

Like many of us Augustine had turned initially to the outer world -- the physical, the objective, the substantial. He thought the answers to life's questions existed in the "hard" reality of tangible entities. Instead he found the visible world a dead end. So he turned to the inner world, the invisible world of mind and soul:

And I turned my thoughts into myself and said, "Who are you?" And I answered, "A [human being]." For see, there is in me both a body and a soul; the one without, the other within. In which of these should I have sought my God, whom I had already sought with my body from earth to heaven . . . But the inner part is the better part; for to it, as both ruler and judge, all these messengers of the senses report the answers of heaven and earth and all the things therein, who said, "We are not God, but [God] made us." My inner [reality] knew these things through the ministry of the outer [reality], and I, the inner [reality], knew all this -- I, the soul, through the senses of my body. I asked the whole frame of earth about my God, and it answered, "I am not [God], but [God] made me" (Augustine 1955, Bk. X, VI, 206-207).

Augustine continued to be puzzled by the seeming contradiction between *his realizing through his sensory experience* the realistic reality of the physical realm and *his realizing through his soul* the meaningful reality of the created order. He pressed the issue of what is physical, and therefore visible, and what is form making, and thereby invisible:

Is not this beauty of form visible to all whose senses are unimpaired? Why, then, does it not say the same things to all? Animals . . . see it but they are unable to interrogate its meaning, because their senses are not endowed with the reason that would enable them to judge the evidence which the senses report. But *[humanity] can interrogate it,* so that "the invisible things of [God] . . . are clearly seen, being understood by the things that are made" (Augustine 1955, Bk. X, VI, 207, emphasis added).

Here he came upon the crux of the issue between what is visible and what is invisible. It is the reality of our "interrogating" our senses! What we perceive always involves more than simple sensations.

We ask "what" something is and we wonder "how" something is. Epistemology involves this issue of "how" we know and "what" we know. And beyond the basic fact of "knowing" lies the ontological issue of the existence and permanence of that knowledge. Finally, we find ourselves asking whether what we "know" about what "exists" really matters ultimately, which is the theological dimension. In short, the neocortex, and more specifically the left hemisphere, always interprets what we observe, making sense of it according to a cosmos of meaning which we ourselves construct but which we assume to be objective.

Augustine turned from the material realm to the primacy of what today we call the cognitive. He replaced the "old" mind of the left brain, which confined itself to the visible and physical, with the "new" mind of the whole cortex, which creates what is seen from what is unseen:

> *only [human beings] understand it who compare the voice received from without with the truth within. For the truth says to me, "Neither heaven nor earth nor anybody is your God." Their very nature tells this to the one who beholds*

*them. "They are a mass, less in part than the whole." Now,
O my soul, you are my better part, and to you I speak; since
you animate the whole mass of your body, giving it life,
whereas no body furnishes life to a body. But your God is
the life of your life (Augustine 1955, Bk. X, VI, 207, emphasis added).*

In exploring that meaning-making reality of the human brain -- its
epistemological dimension -- my purpose is specifically theological. That is, how can we talk about God and the world in a credible
way, a way which is conceptually plausible, empirically identifiable,
and experientially meaningful. To use the combined languages of
empirical science and theological reflection, I am using the human
brain to understand divine being. The brain the neurosciences are
identifying reveals the true reality of our being human.

I am advancing a case for natural theology in an empirical mode.[1]
The brain, with its empirically identified components of cognition,
makes more sense -- and offers more support for belief -- than the
older philosophical understanding of the mind with its faculty of
natural reason. This brain is the "new" mind because we know it is
a brain of three minds. To make my case I review the philosophical and theological traditions of God-talk in The West. I do so because historically "the mind" -- and what it "knows" -- has been burdened with a dualistic split between the way reality appears and the
way reality actually is. The old mind distorts reality, while the new
mind discloses reality.

History of God-Talk: The Old Mind

In the West our understanding of "the mind" -- and what it knows -
- has been burdened with a division between the way things appear
and the way things are. The double mind has distorted reality in
the very process of interpreting reality. It has taken what it observes as final, fixed, permanent. Whatever the left brain has said
about why we act as we act and the reason things appear to be as
they appear has been taken as "fact." In effect, "shovels" exist "be-

cause we need to clean out the chicken shed." The interpretive mind has had the last word about reality.

A review of the history of cognition suggests that the new brain (the neocortex) -- dominated by the left hemisphere yet including the right hemisphere -- has been taken to be "the human mind." I call this mind the "old" rational mind. Whatever the left brain interpreted to be the facts were indeed "the facts." We supposedly lived in an objectively real reality.

The West fostered a tradition in which people reasoned about reason, reflected upon reflection, and have been conscious of consciousness. The left brain did the talking for the new brain. Because of that metaconsciousness, people have inquired about how we conceive of reality and how we converse about that reality.

The Philosophical Tradition

Plato searched for a method to relate reason and reality, logic and life, the sensible statement and the sensory realm. He believed in the existence of an ideal realm from which all else derived. Appearances were shadows of the really real and not reality itself. He assumed a duality between finite matter and eternal essence, and he illustrated what he took to be first principles as they manifested themselves in the sensory world (Burrell 1973, 37-91). He seemed aware intuitively that the left brain did not always know what it was talking about. What was said was always an interpretation of what was being perceived.

The Platonic approach reflected an experiential mode of thinking akin to the right hemisphere. Plato moved from questions such as "What is good?" to the derived question of "The good itself." He reasoned dialectically from the good he knew in appearance to the ideal good he believed to be essential reality. His interpretation included the imaginative leap of right brain process.

Aristotle, however, shifted from that experiential construction of reality to an objective explanation (Burrell 1973, 37-91). He resolved the logical puzzles surrounding ideas such as good, being, and true through "a doctrine of analogy" (Burrell 1973, 68). He identified words and their use as consisting of three types: univocal, equivocal, and analogical.

An univocal word had only one meaning. An equivocal word had conflicting meanings. For instance, a word like "bridge" is equivocal since it could mean an architectural structure spanning a gap between two physical forms, a piece required in a dental procedure, a game of cards, or a metaphorical association between two separate ideas -- all dependent upon the context intended by the speaker.

Between the absolute certainty of univocal words and the impenetrability of equivocal words lay what Aristotle identified as "analogical" words. He assumed that we possess the "ability to grasp relevant similarities" among words and that to which they refer. That grasp of similarities -- common features -- provided the core of his justification for a responsible use of equivocal terms in talking about reality. It is now known as "the principle of focal meaning" (Burrell 1973, 75).

According to this logic, those instances of focal meaning identified an underlying order. But we were dependent on the "instances" to provide clues to that substance. The formal order could not be known directly, only indirectly in and through the particular. Not only did what the left brain say reflect the elusiveness of what it observed, but even more what it said assumed an objective referent to the interpretive statement. Aristotle shifted the use of language from the dialectic of right-left brain collaboration to the static context of arithmetic (Burrell 1973, 77), which characterizes left brain process.

In effect, Plato proceeded dialectically. It was as though he knew implicitly that the left brain was interpreting input from the whole brain, unlike split brain patient Paul. In contrast, Aristotle utilized analogies which gave priority to left brain explanation.

However, the consequence of the assumption of a duality about reality -- whether Platonic experience or Aristotelian analogy -- made left brain process dominant. The rationalistic objective metaphysics reigned supreme in classic western thought.

The human brain was thought to mirror reality. Its concepts were merely the "internal representations of external reality" (Lakoff 1987, 370-373). Reality, thereby, consisted of entities with fixed, shared, essential, and eternal properties.

The Theological Tradition

Thomas Aquinas built upon the duality of the Platonic tradition and the objectivism of the Aristotelian tradition. The approach of analogy of being assumed a similarity between the sensory world and the spiritual realm. Thomas recognized that analogical similarity was a matter of the way language was used and not a matter of objective reality -- in principle, something which "qualitatively" distinguished between what we know only in part in the sensory realm and what we cannot know but is perfectly present in spiritual reality. He avoided the static "logic of analogy" by systematically pursuing analogical thinking and analogical expressions (Burrell 1973, 122).

The Thomists, however, characterized the similarity between the sensory and the spiritual by mathematical proportionality. In principle, the two spheres were distinguished "quantitatively," that is, in terms of a mathematical ratio between what was imperfectly known -- in us and by us -- yet was perfectly known -- in God and of God. That objective view found its fullest expression in the gothic edifice of Scholastic construction. Humanity, so the belief went, could move rationally from the sensory world of objects to the spiritual realm of subjects, and, finally, to the transcendent realm of Being Itself or God.

From the Greeks through the Scholastics, including Aquinas, therefore, the use of analogy, analogy of being, and analogical thinking characterized the way in which believers talked about

God. The old rational mind reflected the eternal mind in a way which was mathematically proportional, which meant in a way which was precise, objective, substantial and permanent.

A shift came with the Reformers. They were skeptical about the ontological assumption that God could be known through the orderly structure of the universe itself. Natural knowledge acquired by the philosophic method could never give true knowledge of God (Mondin 1968, 104). They dismissed objective knowability, which meant intelligibility.

The principle of knowing was clear: *sola fide, by faith alone! Expressions of God were expressions of faith. Such expressions could not be identified with sensory reality, even analogically. The Reformers called into question every literal interpretation of nature.*

In the tradition of the Reformers, Church theologian Karl Barth argued against analogy of being on the basis of analogy of faith (Mondin 1968, 147-173). Thus, theologian Sallie McFague (1982) suggests that metaphorical God-talk is more Protestant and analogical God-talk is more Catholic. By this she means that metaphor assumes and expresses no necessary relationship between the things referred to, whereas analogy assumes and expresses some necessary similarity. The Catholic heritage has always allowed a place for natural theology along side of revealed theology (Tracy 1983). In contrast, the Protestant heritage has viewed such continuity between creation and Creator as heresy. There is no connection, it claims. At best creation ex nihilo allows only for creation in the image or likeness of God.

Despite crucial differences between Catholic Substance and Protestant Principle, philosophical theologian Paul Tillich made the classic statement of a natural theology: God is not a being but Being Itself (Tillich 1951, 235ff). As he put it, his own use of symbolic knowledge meant "exactly what St. Thomas means with analogia entis" (quoted by Mondin 1968, 144). Here is the pinnacle of a natural philosophical approach to understanding what matters most in, to, and for the universe as we know it. "[B]ecause everything participates in being-itself . . .[t]he <u>analogia entis</u> gives us our only justification of speaking at all about God" (Tillich 1951, 239-240). As the Power of Being Itself, God manifests God in every part of being.

More recently, philosopher Charles Hartshorne (1967), theologian John Cobb (1965), and others have developed a natural theology based on the process metaphysics of Alfred North Whitehead. They have attempted to overcome the metaphysical limitations in the traditional world views (Young, 1987). Specifically, that means the dualistic view of Plato, the substantialistic view based of Aristotle, the mechanistic view stemming from Newton, and the Cartesian view which assumed a disjuncture between mind and body. Process philosophy is "entirely open," Cobb attests (1977, 32), to an analogical orientation which acknowledges a continuity between the human, the natural, and the physical.

Experiential Realism: The New Mind

God-talk, consequently, includes and requires both metaphorical and analogical uses of language. In fact, all language is metaphorical, according to linguist George Lakoff and philosopher Mark Johnson (Lakoff and Johnson 1980; Lakoff 1987). In contrast to the classical view of cognition as propositional or left brain, new evidence shifts our understanding from traditional objectivism to an experiential realism or more whole brain.

In this revised view of the mind, cognition consists of the following attributes:

> (1) is embodied, which means it arises out of bodily experience and makes sense primarily in terms of bodily experience. The core of our conceptual systems is grounded directly in what we perceive, in bodily movement, and in experience which is both physical and social;

(2) is imaginative, which means that concepts not grounded directly in experience go beyond literal mirroring or representing external reality in that they employ "metaphor, metonym [that is, understanding the whole in terms of a part], and mental imagery" -- all of which are more than we can see and feel;

(3) possesses gestalt properties, an overall structure which is other than merely putting together individual conceptual building blocks according to general rules of association; and

(4) has an ecological structure which "depends on the overall structure of the conceptual system and on what the concepts mean." Thought, then, can be described as using cognitive models rather than just mechanically manipulating abstract symbols (Lakoff 1987, xiv-xv).

This evidence contradicts the rationalistic metaphysics of western thought. Reality does not consist of entities which feature fixed, essential, and common properties. People make sense of things in many ways (Lakoff 1987), 119) -- whether that be family relationships (Lakoff 1987, 22-24); colors (Lakoff 1987, 24-30); linguistic categories (Lakoff 1987, 58-67); biological groupings (Lakoff 1987, 118-121; Berlin 1978); or anger, lust, and rape (Lakoff 1987, 380-415). The representation of reality always includes those engaging in the act of cognition itself.

In brief, the human brain does not mirror nature nor are concepts merely "internal representations of external reality" (Lakoff 1987, 370-373). Because meaning and truth are based on an understanding of the cultural context in which they arise, categories are never mutually exclusive nor permanently objective (Lakoff 1987, 202). There is no such thing as "mind-free reality" (Lakoff 1987, 212). Knowledge clusters at a basic level which depends upon the following: a) fast identification of similarly perceived shapes and a single mental image reflecting an entire category, b) motor actions used in interacting with other members of the category, c) the most commonly used and contextually neutral form of communicating the category, and d) an organization of knowledge which takes into account the most attributes of members of the particular category (Lakoff 1987, 46-47).

These levels of the organization of knowledge -- the superordinate, the basic, and the subordinate -- can be illustrated with two taxonomic hierarchies, one involving the category "animal" and the other the category "furniture" (Lakoff 1987, 46):

Cognition According to Experiential Realism

Superordinate Level:	animal	furniture
Basic Level:	dog	chair
Subordinate Level:	retriever	rocker

The categories "animal" and "furniture" are the most abstract -- the superordinate level. The categories "retriever" and rocker" add virtually no additional information to the basic level of "dog" and "chair." The basic level, therefore, is literally "basic" because it provides the most information about a category.

Take the criteria of knowledge at the basic level I cited above and apply it to the taxonomic hierarchies of what constitutes "dog" and "chair." Each has a concreteness -- an "[o]verall perceived shape; [a] single mental image; [which permits] fast identification" of whether something is a "dog" or a "chair." Each enables us to use similar behaviors -- motor action programs -- to relate to the members of the category as a "dog" or a "chair." Each is referred to in the "[s]hortest, most commonly used and contextually neutral words, first learned by children and first" to be used in a stable way in speech -- someone saying to a young child as he or she points to a dog, "dog" or "doggie," or similarly pointing to a chair and saying "chair." Each object -- dog or chair -- possesses the "[m]ost attributes of category members . . . stored at this level" (Lakoff 1987, 46-47).

The categories "dog" and "chair" are generalizations based upon experiences of people seeing particular dogs such as a "retriever" and particular chairs such as a "rocker." Because the particulars are so specific they do not add enough information to enable us to organize more information beyond what we first learned in identifying members of these categories. Such specifics as "retriever" and "rocker," however, enable us to generalize -- to imagine a pattern or category -- about such particulars, with the result that the categories "dog" and "chair" are located at the basic level of cognition.

Linguist Eleanor Rosch and her associates (Rosch and Lloyd 1978) have established that we organize knowledge primarily according to cue validity. Cue validity consists of two features: (a) cognitive economy, or gaining as much information about the environment as possible while conserving limited resources, and (b) the world perceived as a highly correlational structure (Rosch 1978, 27-48). Both superordinate and subordinate categories exhibit low cue validity. Basic level abstraction maximizes both cue validity and category resemblance in terms of what are known as representative examples (exemplars) or prototypes. The dome of St. Sophia is a prototype of Byzantine architecture, as the spire of Chartres is a prototype of Medieval architecture.

To clarify the difference between classical cognition and empirical cognitivism, especially as these views of knowledge apply to belief or theology, I contrast their assumptions. (A detailed discussion of specific differences between, say, Platonic assumptions and Aristotelian assumptions or Reformed Protestant assumptions and Roman Catholic assumptions is beyond the scope of this analysis.) Consider a taxonomic hierarchy of classical objectivism first:

Classical Objectivism

<u>philosophical theological</u>

(abstract/objective)

Superordinate Level:	Reality-Essences	Spiritual-Deity

Being Itself

Basic Level:	proportional similarities
Subordinate Level:	Deceptive Appearances

Platonic   Protestant *sola fide*

Sensory Reality

Aristotelian   Catholic *analogia entis*

I suggest that in the classical tradition of the West, the concept of Being Itself comes at the superordinate level. It is the most over-arching, whether in the philosophical domain and its use of "Reality" or "Essences" or in the theological domain with its use of "Spiritual" or "Deity." These categories allow no perceptual experience, no sensory data upon which to imagine and thereby create a base of information. Language resources are stretched -- taxed -- to give meaning to the categories.

The subordinate level is perceptual and experiential. However, physical reality is understood in the most general way and with quite different understandings. From Platonic and Protestant perspectives the sensory domain is deceptive, which is why metaphor and faith, respectively, are needed in knowing the really real. From Aristotelian and Roman Catholic perspectives the sensory reality is disclosive, which is why analogy between what is visible and what is invisible makes knowledge of the really real possible. However, in each instance the physical realm adds virtually no information which is not available at the basic level of proportional dissimilarities or similarities. The hierarchy assumes a rational structure to the universe, a dualistic distinction between the sensory world and eternal essence or God. Deceptive appearance requires a metaphorical leap so that proportional similarity is understood qualitatively, while sensory reality is an analogical step so that proportional similarity is quantitative.

I suggest a different taxonomy of knowledge based on the new cognitivism:

The New Cognitivism

	linguistic	theological
	(truth as constellational/cultural)	
Superordinate Level:	generalizations	values & beliefs
Basic Level:	prototypical effects	
	bodily/imaginative	analogical expressions
Subordinate Level:	specific instances	

Whether we are dealing with language or theology, knowledge consists of constellations of cultural perceptions. Truth, therefore, is never absolute, objective, and eternal. At the superordinate level, we generalize and articulate values and beliefs. Because these represent abstract information, they convey the least amount of knowledge. Specific instances are located at the subordinate level because they are specific and add little to that which is known at the basic level. The basic level, therefore, includes prototypical effects, constellations of perception and patterns. In the linguistic realm, these constellations come from bodily perception and leaps of imagination (Johnson 1987), while in the theological realm, these prototypical effects include metaphorical-analogical expressions such as God's body, or God as mother, lover, friend (McFague 1987).

With this background about the nature of cognition -- objective essence or experiential realism -- I add two other hierarchies. These hierarchies suggest how empirical and philosophical modes of natural theology might be viewed in a manner parallel to and clarified by the approach to knowledge based on perceived similarities which give rise to dimensional structures.

Natural Theology

	empirical-existential	philosophical
Superordinate Level:	meaning/God	divine intuition/above thought
Basic Level:	human brain:	experience as:
	empirical-existential	participatory-valuational
Subordinate Level:	individual brains	relativities

The basic level includes categories which best represent "the correlational structure of the environment" (Rosch 1978). For our discussion, "meaning/God" and "divine intuition/above thought" may be regarded as superordinate categories. The categories "human brain" and "experience" are concepts at the basic level. The "brain" may be perceived empirically or existentially. Similarly, "experience" may be perceived experientially or cognitively. "Individual brains" with their own idiosyncratic features and "relativities" are located at the subordinate level and do not add to what is available at the basic level.

This new cognitivism recognizes there is no one way to frame a situation or define a category (Lakoff 1987, 200). We organize what we know by means of idealized models, or prototype effects. Best-fit examples or representations of a category are identified. These arise from the interactions between a given schema with other schema in the system (Lakoff 1987, 70). Because we construct reality from prototypical exemplars and exemplars possess only "a degree of prototypicality" (Lakoff 1987, 44), we deal with the world as we understand it and not with the "world as it is" apart from us (Lakoff 1987, 212).

Rational cognition thereby is anchored in the abstract, the disembodied, and the literal, while natural cognition is centered in the bodily and the imaginative (Lakoff 1987, 370-373; Johnson 1987). The traditional view of what is "natural," "logical," and "cognitive" has been too narrow, based as it has on a structure of abstract and absolute principles (Rumelhart et al 1986; Holyoak 1987; Pribram

1987). Our current view of what is "natural" or "cognitive" (Gardner 1985², calls for a wider cognitivism, a view of "natural" informed by the empirical.

The old view of mind no longer reflects what we know and how we think. A new view of mind is emerging. Process thought reflects that new mind in a philosophical approach, but it is the brain sciences which are identifying that new mind empirically.

Mind As Bridge

A superfical view of what is happening in the brain sciences could be characterized as a move downward from psyche to soma, from mind to brain, from spirit to matter. The dramatic attention to the chemical make-up of the brain as "the hardware of consciousness" (Hooper and Teresi [1986] 1987) supports that impression. In efforts to cope with various forms of mental dysfunction and mental illness, scientists have turned increasingly to biopsychological and psychopharmacological processes (Snyder 1974). For instance, chemical imbalance contributes to severe depression and so is treated medically. Instead of exploring how a person feels or thinks, effort is directed to how the brain operates biochemically. Quite simply, the focus marks a shift from "oppressive beliefs" and "troubled minds" to "broken brains" (Andreasen 1985). The evidence is clear: genetic, biochemical, and neurological factors contribute to disturbed behavior (Tanguay 1985).

A closer look, however, reveals a more complex picture (Ashbrook 1987a). Biological intervention by itself is not enough. We need think only of the disillusionment surrounding the deinstitutionalization of the mentally ill by putting them back into the community. Families, support networks, social conditions, interpretive frames of meaning affect our lives as much as chemistry. These enhance or restrict what is done medically.

Competence in the laboratory sciences is no substitute for an inability to talk with patients as human beings, according to psychiatrist Roy Menninger. He worries about the psychiatric con-

centration on the drug cabinet in a misguided effort to find a
magic pill for patient pain (Grossman 1987). A multidimensional
approach to human pain takes into account the complexities of
body-mind interaction: cultural beliefs, biological brains, social
conditions, and individual minds.

The Change In How We View Ourselves

Notions that mind is not separate from body nor body from mind
are bringing changes in the way we understand ourselves.

In efforts to understand how cultural values and beliefs are
mapped onto the brain, part of psychology has been moving upward from soma as physical to psyche as cognitive. Traditional distinctions such as mind-body or matter-spirit no longer fit the empirical data. Researcher Howard Gardner interprets this
phenomenon as the cognitive revolution. For him and others, it
has become "the mind's new science" (Gardner 1985).

Until the last two decades we have been limited in understanding
the connection between soma and psyche, between feeling and
thought, and between the brain and belief. Neurologist Oliver
Sacks hints at that difficulty in describing the trauma of breaking
his leg. When he lost a sense of his leg, he lost a clear sense of
himself (Sacks [1984] 1987a).

During his recovery, Sacks returned to a detailed reading of the
great English neurologist Sir Henry Head who worked in the early
part of this century. In writing of *Aphasia* (and the loss of the
ability to speak, which usually goes with paralysis of the right side
of the body), Head described a doubleness in experience. Two
modes of thought or two realms of reality seemed joined in learning to talk and walk again.

There was the domain of analysis, of science, of neurology -- as
suggested by such words as "sequence," "series," "complex procedures," all of which needed to be mobilized with "chronological ex-
actitude" if a patient were to regain those capacities. It was a

mechanical, step-by-step, self-conscious, deliberate procedure. Then there was the domain of the poetic, expressed in words like "completeness," "wholeness," "perfection," and "melody." This was imaginative, rhythmic, all-at-once, unthinking, spontaneous movement.

Sacks recalled his father, who had been Head's resident in those early years, saying of Head: "He was the most rigorous of scientists, but he was a poet too. He *felt* the music of movement and speech, but as a neurologist he could not *explain* it." What Sacks came to realize, and what the description of Head revealed, is clear: a mechanical approach to healing misses the "human" dimension of both emotional *and* physical brokenness. What mattered in a patient's recovery was vivid natural experience unspoiled by abstract conceptualization (Sachs [1984] 1987a, 198-204). To "think about" walking only made matters worse. The patient had to find his or her own "unthinking" sense of movement.

One day Sachs' physiotherapist threw him into the swimming pool. Miraculously, his leg, with its "natural" ability to move, suddenly returned to its proper place in the scheme of things. Without "thinking," Sachs once again found himself moving with the rhythmic wholeness he had possessed before his injury. His own fearfully mechanical approach to recovery had impeded his progress. Once he moved naturally -- poetically, in Head's word -- he again found his leg and "himself."

We are on the threshold of a revolution in our approach to the body and belief. The poetic, aesthetic, or religious traditions have always known that inner reality (Ornstein [1972, 1977] 1986), even if they have been limited in their ability to explain the physical face of personal meaning, and even though they have expressed it in cathedrals like St. Sophia and Chartres as I describe above.

In reflecting upon his own experience of himself, for instance, Augustine voiced the doubleness to which Head alluded: "I do not myself grasp all that I am. Thus the mind is too narrow to contain itself. But where can that part be which it does not contain" (Augustine 1955, Bk. X, VIII, 210)? Sach's music beyond mechanism points toward an unanticipated resolution of the dualism between mind and body, what in religious language we call spirit and matter.

The cognitive revolution is returning "mind" to a substantial place in our understanding of ourselves and how we function. Popular books are heralding the unity of body and mind (cf. Benson 1975, 1979, 1984; Siegel 1986; Borysenko 1987). No longer can we view ourselves -- and even other mammals -- as passive objects, mechanical organisms, to be manipulated chemically with no attention to the experiential reality which is expressed in and through the physical. We know the crucial role the limbic system plays in that unity. It is the bodily basis of all that we feel, imagine, and about which we reason (Rossi 1986; see also Johnson 1987).

Mind is neither its own origin nor its own destiny. As brain, the concept *mind* gives "human" meaning to its biological origin, integrating nature and nurture. As brain, the concept *mind* gives "human" meaning to the evolutionary matrix out of which both itself and culture have emerged. As brain, the concept *mind* gives "human" meaning to the universe in which it finds itself, thereby embodying the "human" meaning of divine purpose.

The brain constructs a reasonable view of reality, as split brain patient Paul demonstrated. To have a brain and to give a reasonable explanation of the world are one and the same reality. To have a brain is to be a co-creator of what matters most in human life.

Except in conditions which suspend or negate its natural functioning, the brain does not work in isolation from the world. We are part of, and we shape, universes of influence -- social, cultural, cosmic. We live in a contextual universe, a universe of meaning which we create as much as find. Cognitive psychologist Urich Neisser describes that relationship between cognition and reality with a cleverly concise statement:

> No choice is ever free of the information on which it is based. Nevertheless, that information is selected by the chooser. . . . On the other hand, no choice is ever determined by the environment directly. Still, that environment supplies the information the chooser will use (Neisser 1976, 182).

In other words, mind must be understood as semi-autonomous in terms of the environment. It is "semi" in the sense that the neocortex is always processing information from both the old cortex and what it observes in the environment. Therefore it is not creating something out of nothing.

Mind is "autonomous" in that its associations, connections, gestalts go beyond sensory input. It combines sensory input in novel ways in the association cortex. The cerebral cortex transforms the regularities of the reptilian and the mammalian brains into emergent mental re-presentations. The results are what the brain of three minds takes to be real and right, or true.

These cognitive maps express emotional convictions about how the world is put together. The reptilian and mammalian brains do not displace the new brain nor does the new brain displace the older brains. In effect, the concept *mind* constitutes the *human* meaning of the physical brain (Ashbrook 1984b).

The Emergent Mind

Put this way, we can approach cognition as an emergent phenomenon. Mind comes out of nature and does not function apart from nature. Mind shapes the physical world even as the physical world shapes mind.

The cognitive -- or mental to use the more conventional word -- bridges what we take to be physical and what we regard as human.

Matter and meaning are each aspects of biochemical activity. Molecular biology and brain studies point to "the inseparability or oneness of the reality designed by the two domains called 'life' and 'matter' and the two domains called 'mind' and 'matter'" (Burhoe 1981, 126). Their features and reaches are shaped by the fields of influence -- contexts -- in which they are located and with which they interact. The brain, as *human* matter, both reflects the historical reality of the world and shapes that reality on the basis of its own input, including its reptilian and mammalian input. We integrate our cultural contexts and our genetic inheritances into the living realities which we all are (Trevarthen 1986).

At the loose interface between physical data and vivid personal experience -- that nonphysical yet imaginable space which Gordon Rattray Taylor (1979) defines as mind -- we find clues to the human meaning of our human presence in a physical universe (Sperry 1977; 1982). Those clues consist of "such fancy trimmings as a sense of identity, a sense of humor or a sense of deity" (Taylor 1979, 17-19). These trimmings reflect core features of our brain: our identity as persons; our capacity for perspective through humor; and the nature of the contextual universe in which we locate ourselves or what in religious language we call God. We are part of "a single natural system" (Burhoe 1981, 82, 74-75).

Somewhat unexpectedly, the cognitive revolution is contributing to the pivotal notion of mind (Gardner 1985). Instead of referring to mind per se, the mind's new science focuses on the centrality of mental representations. We con-ceive an objective world by joining together into one mental representation: (i) our bodily experience, (ii) the realism of our perceptions, and (iii) the synthesis of our imagination. A set of constructs -- variously labelled as schemas, images, rules, frames, transformations -- is used to explain phenomena. These phenomena range from what we see, to understanding stories, to what I call "belief," which is the configuration of assumptions we make about reality.

I view this breakthrough in making sense of human life as a wider view of cognition than the older dualistic view of mind distinct from body. This more natural cognition incorporates physical explanations at the level of the neuronal brain, socio-psychological explanations at the level of the socio-cultural mind (Gardner 1985, 383), and spiritual explanations at the level of the soul.

Left brain cognition follows the rules of formal logic. Its information comes from what it observes. It uses language in a way which creates a second-order vocabulary. That is, its vocabulary is less about actual events and objects and more about whether statements are consistent or inconsistent (Gardner 1985, 385). Again, split brain Paul's explanation about the shovel and the shed illustrates the way we create consistency by providing a rationale which makes the puzzling sensible. We make sense of life through the way we interpret life. It is the left brain's logic which gives the appearance of an objective reality.

In contrast, right brain cognition works according to a situational logic. Its information arises from an imaginative construction of patterns or wholes. These mosaics of what is meaningful result from what can be described as simultaneous, distributed, and parallel processing. Though it never works independently of left brain input, especially in the frontal area, the right brain functions in a way that falls "into patterns with huge numbers of interconnections and a minimum of formal symbolic processing" (DeAngelis 1987; Rumelhart et al [1986] 1987; cf. Pribram 1986). Its ability seems to be based on "the *pars-pro-toto* principle, that is, the immediate recognition of a totality on the basis of *one* essential detail" (Watzlawick 1978, 69-73). Everything is there -- all at once, by a leap of imagination. We see, according to MacLean, "archetypes," partial representations which we take for the whole (Hooper and Teresi [1986] 1987, 47).

Pars-pro-toto is a way of seeing things obliquely -- not looking at an object or event straight on or with a direct studied look but rather from a glancing, off centered view. This may be similar to "seeing through a glass darkly" (1 Corinthians 13:12). And it may be exactly the way that part of the brain has to operate later on in order to make symbolic connections possible through images which are seen, though they are not seen in an objective or physical sense.

Holographic Order

Research scientists such as Karl Pribram identify this phenomenon of the oblique imaging of the whole as "the holographic paradigm" (Wilber 1985; Pribram 1985; Pribram 1986, 514). We do not "see" objects directly, rather we "construct" objects as when we listen to music from two stereo speakers so balanced that the sound seems to come from a point midway between them (Wilber 1985, 9).

Holography is a form of optical storage in which each individual section (part) of a photographic plate contains the image of the whole picture in condensed form. If you take a holographic picture of a person, for instance, and cut a section out of the person's head, and then enlarge that section to the original size of the picture, you do not get a big head but rather the whole person (Wilber 1985, 2).

Belief patterns are basically holographic. When theologians talk about unity-in-diversity, therefore, they are saying that the whole is in the part; and when they speak of diversity-in-unity, they are indicating that the part contains the whole. Any and every part of the hologram reconstructs the whole image.

From research and reflection on the precise mathematical holographic transformations of waves of information, which are distributed over the whole of the photographic film, into whole images, Pribram speculates about the classic dichotomy between the physical and the mental (Pribram 1986; 1985). He rejects the mentalist who gives the weight of evidence to experience and phenomenology, as he rejects the materialist who gives the weight of evidence to "the contents of the experience" and the physical. For him, "structure" constitutes both mind and brain in that each proceeds in a different direction in conceptualizing and realizing systems of information (Pribram 1986, 512). The brain does not, according to him, organize input gained from the physical world through the senses and from this "constructs mental properties." Instead, and this is the astonishing speculation: "Mental properties are the pervasive organizing principles of the universe, which includes the brain" (Pribram 1985, 29-30).

Mind reflects the basic structure of the universe. It is the relationships which exist among the many observations which are cognitive and thereby mental phenomena. This leads Pribram to suggest that "[p]erhaps the very fundamental properties of the universe are therefore mental and not material" (Pribram 1985, 29). Order itself constitutes the really real and not the components which make up order. In theological language that has been called "Logos." In the beginning is Word!

The question becomes whether mind and cognition are "emergents or expressions of some basic ordering principle" (Pribram 1985, 33-34). If "emergent" from nature, then mind evolves from brain and brain evolves from matter and matter means separate particles of dust. If "expressions" of nature, then mind reveals a basic undivided, whole, implicit universe of imaged relationships. Then the separate "entities" which we observe in ordinary time and space are images which we "read out" from each part which has access to the whole even as the whole is present in each part.

A photographic lens focuses, objectifies, and sharpens boundaries between parts of any scene. It functions in a left brain step-by-step manner. In contrast, holographic operations are distributed, implicit, unbounded, and holistic. These operate in a right brain all-at-once way which draws directly upon the subsymbolic parallel distributed process of the limbic system. Our senses "make sense" of reality "by tuning in (and out) selective portions of this [holographic] domain" (Pribram 1986, 517-518).

Understood this way, the brain becomes an analyzer and transformer of energy and relationships. Reality consists of the imaged configurations of energy systems rather than their raw objective stimuli. Only the ordinary world of experience is made up of physical matter. Real reality is "neither material nor mental, but neutral . . . [an] informational structure" which organizes energy (Pribram 1986, 512).

As Gardner put the issue of this wider form of cognition, we do not approach the "more complex and belief-tainted processes such as classification of ontological domains or judgments concerning rival courses of action . . . in a manner that can be characterized as logical or rational or that entail step-by-step symbolic processing" (Gardner 1985, 385). What we believe to be true, what we take to be right, what we decide is the best way to proceed in a specific situation all require a patterning of reality which involves something other than a logical progression. Instead, we use biases, images, hunches, vague patterns, yes, and beliefs as well. In my mind this wider cognition describes what faith is and how faith functions.

For me, faith is the experiential anchoring of what matters most in life. It appears in the old brain, below the conscious level of the two hemispheres. That bodily sense of reality then gets voiced in terms of what we believe. As *The Letter to the Hebrews* puts it, "faith is the assurance of things hoped for, the conviction of things not seen" (Hebrews 11:1 RSV). "Assurance" and "conviction" about what matters are right brain responses to limbic activity in the service of survival of the self and continuity of the species. Belief thereby is a transformation of biological experience into left brain explanations.

The formal categories of the left brain tend to take on permanence. It is as though these categories of "what's there" -- objects, experiences, and events, or even ourselves, the world, and God -- actually exist as objective "entities" so that when we think about them, our mind is "mirroring" the "entity" in the external world. But in viewing our categories as existing independently of ourselves we fail to take account of the fact that these perceptions are always "messy, intuitive, [and] subject to subjective representations" (Gardner 1985, 380, 386).

These intuitive representations reflect right brain and limbic decision-making as to what is perceived and whether that is desirable or undesirable, to be approached or avoided, to be sought or fought. Here in the dim messiness of life we find the crucial human issues. These issues are "the role of the surrounding context, the affective aspects of experience, and the effects of cultural and historical factors" on how we act (Gardner 1985, 387). Everything we think or feel exists in a context of meaning which we construct based upon bodily experience and the imaginative use of reason (Johnson 1987; Lakoff 1987).

Subsymbolic Reality

Some scientists are now calling this process "the *subsymbolic paradigm*." That means "the most powerful level of description of cognitive systems is hypothesized to be lower than the level that is naturally described by symbol manipulation" (Rumelhart et al [1986] 1987, Vol. 1, 195), or what we ordinarily think of as language. For all the power of the symbolic-sequential capability of our left hemisphere, it is the subsymbolic activity of our total cortex which accounts more adequately and accurately for what we know and how we know it. The left brain simply does not function without the subsymbolic activity of the rest of the brain, nor does the rest of the brain function without the symbolic activity of the left and right hemispheres.

In other words, left brain logic approaches reality in terms of a symbolic paradigm. The symbolic paradigm is restricted to the new brain and more especially to its rational mind, though it is important to remember the intuitive right brain creates the symbolic pattern. I suggest this process of abstracting realistic features from immediate experience contributes to the dualistic distinction between an objective physical world and a subjective phenomenal realm.

The new data of brain research directs us toward an approach to reality more in terms of a subsymbolic paradigm. The approach gives greater weight to natural processes in meaning-making, what are technically known as category construction and definitional classification (Lakoff 1987, Johnson 1987): what features constitute "an object" and how is that object distinguished from all other objects? These natural processes operate at every level of brain organization, and, by so doing, are identified as massively parallel and widely distributed in both what is represented and how it is controlled. The action combines memory *and* novel associations of memories. This mindful brain makes us different from the machine-like left hemisphere and the animal-like (nonconscious) right hemisphere. We construct a world -- the realism of the symbolic paradigm -- in terms of our subsymbolic experience.

We are better than machines (Rumelhardt et al [1986] 1987, Vol. 1, 3) at "perceiving objects in natural scenes." We are quicker at noting relationships. We more easily understand commands and retrieve "contextually appropriate information from memory." We make plans and carry them out more effectively than even the most sophisticated computer. In essence, we are "smarter than today's computers."

Our brain is better suited to deal with tasks which require "the simultaneous consideration of many pieces of information or constraints," since every constraint may be vague, ambiguous, and inadequately specified. Furthermore, "most everyday situations cannot be rigidly assigned to just a single" frame of reference or schemata of meaning (Rumelhardt et al [1986] 1987, Vol. 1, 9). This kind of common sense complexity requires a grasp of the context in which we act, and it is precisely the context which is of our own making.

We are better than animals at sequential symbolic processing. In the past we have called this "rationality" our capacity to imagine, to think, to plan, to implement, to evaluate in conscious ways. It points to the higher-ordering processing in which we engage -- the macrostructures of meaning. There is no way our cultural heritage, with its technology and its artistry, can be explained simply on the basis of genetics alone (Burhoe 1981; 1987). Unlike other animals we can pass on to future generations accumulated information about the past. That is why so much of our experience consists of what we learn instead of what is instinctual.

According to the mythical interpretations of our origin in *The Book of Genesis*, we are breathing dust (Genesis 2:7). We embody all that is and is to be, created, as the phrase has it, "in the image and likeness" of that Reality which is and will be what it will be (Genesis 1:27, Exodus 3:14). Undoubtedly, this capacity to order "Order" -- to have dominion over everything (Genesis 1:28b) by "naming" it (Genesis 2:19-20) and thereby objectifying it -- reflects the origin of the Psalmist's joyful song:

> When I look at thy heavens, the work of thy fingers,
>   the moon and the stars which thou hast established,
> what [are we] that thou art mindful of [us],
>   and [our children] that thou dost care for [them]?
>
> Yet thou hast made [us] little less than God,
>   and dost crown [us] with glory and honor.
> Thou hast given [us] dominion over the works of thy hands;
>   thou hast put all things under [our] feet,
> all sheep and oxen,
>   and also the beasts of the field,
> the birds of the air, and the fish of the sea,
>   whatever passes along the paths of the sea.

However, in singing of the workings of this higher-order processing of the neocortex, the Psalmist ends as he began -- with a recognition of the larger universe in which his brain and ours exists:

> O Lord, our Lord,
> how majestic is thy name in all the earth!
>   (Psalm 8 RSV)

In effect, logic is embedded in a distributed, parallel, simultaneous, contextual network of meaning (Rumelhardt et al [1986] 1987, Vol. 2, 548). I take this subsymbolic, microstructure of meaning, to consist of "observed regularities." I characterize those regularities as belief patterns.

Language is metaphorical (Lakoff and Johnson 1980), an imaginative creation based on visceral experience and visual perception (Johnson 1987; Lakoff 1987). Words are not permanent, substantial, independent entities; they are finite, subjective configurations of reasonable sensibilities. In fact, the right brain remains the more basic agency of human activity by virtue of its broad associations and ready connections with the emotive limbic system (Burhoe 1987).

Figurative and denotative languages -- the poetic and the mechanical, the religious and the scientific, the metaphorical and the analogical -- are not different types of meaning arising from different brain processes. Instead, I submit that what is suggestive and what is exact, what is psyche and what is soma, what is purposeful and what is physical, what is mind and what is brain are "coarse categories describing the nature of the meanings synthesized" by parallel distributed processing networks (Rumelhardt et al [1986] 1987, Vol. 2, 550). This is how and why the cognitive revolution is carrying us into a deeper realm of mental representation than the enlightenment of The Age of Reason ever suspected.

Scientists insist we are a long way from connecting our more abstract networks with particular brain structures" (Rumelhardt et al [1986] 1987, Vol. 2, 552). Along with an aggressive optimism about what they can accomplish -- given time and resources -- most researchers voice the kind of modesty which Alan Gevins, director of the EEG Systems Laboratory in San Francisco, did:

> As scientists we sometimes get very arrogant about all
> our fancy toys. But we're like cavemen when it comes to
> understanding anything fundamental about the relation-

ship between the mind and the brain. If you try to imagine what astronomy was like before the invention of the telescope or microbiology before the microscope ... well, that's where we are in brain science (Hooper and Teresi [1986] 1987, 144).

Even so, it is evident that our left brain's reasoning capacity is an interpretation of our right brain's meaning-making sensibility. Despite that vigilance, our right brain's responsiveness to the felt-meaning of our environment continues to be primary. Whole brain processing is more basic than half brain activity (Levy 1985b). Objective, as well as ordinary, consciousness carries on with all the exact representational which assumes that the maps we make in our heads correspond to the territory in which we find ourselves. But maps are never the territory (Korzybski 1933; Hooper and Teresi [1986] 1987, 103-104). Increasingly, we are recognizing that no amount of human mastery can dispel the cosmic mystery which we incarnate. Our three pound universe reveals an integrated and integrating reality, a higher-order processing of lower level chaos (cf. Genesis 1-3).

Because we now recognize the importance of the older brain, we are discovering the new mind -- the mind of many dimensions. The old logical brain has turned out to be a figment of our rationalized imagination. The new mind at last makes faith sensible, for faith is

> the conviction of things not seen ... so that what is seen was made out of things which do not appear.
> (Hebrews 11: 1,3 RSV)

NOTES

1. Empirical theology in America has been primarily interested in the phenomenological description of personal and social experience (Meland 1969; Dean 1986; Frankenberry 1987) rather

than the narrower focus of the brain sciences which I am intending for the empirical.

2. Lakoff identifies cognitive science as a field which brings together psychology, linguistics, anthropology, philosophy, and computer science in seeking detailed answers to such questions as: "What is reason? How do we make sense of our experience? What is a conceptual system and how is it organized? Do all people use the same conceptual system? If so, what is that system? If not, exactly what is there that is common to the way all human beings think? (Lakoff 1987, xi). Gardner (1985) adds artificial intelligence and neuroscience to the field.

CHAPTER SIX

WONDROUSLY MADE

Yahweh, what variety you have created . . .
You give breath, fresh life begins,
you keep renewing the world.
(Psalm 104:24, 30-31a JB)

we import a secret and hidden wisdom of God,
which God decreed before the ages
for our glorification . . .
as it is written,
"What no eye has seen
nor ear heard,
not the heart conceive,
what God has prepared
for those who love [God],"

God has revealed to us
through the Spirit.
For the Spirit searches everything,
even the depths of God.
(1 Corinthians 2:7-19 RSV)

The concept of mind, as the human aspects of brain, directs our attention downward into the organized regularities of the reptilian-mammalian levels and equally encourages us to turn outward toward the emergent aspects of human purposes. The royal road toward understanding how culture is mapped onto brains, as cognitive scientist Howard Gardner puts it, is the representational level (Gardner 1985, 390-391). The new mind makes belief more credible.

Mother Julian lived as a fourteenth century recluse in Norwich, England (1342-1416). In describing her mystical "shewings" (or visions), she voiced the experience of the Middle Ages with special clarity:

> Whether our urge is to know God or to know our own soul matters little: both are good and true. . . .Our substance and sensuality together are rightly named our soul, because they are united by God . . .we can never attain to the full knowledge of God until we have first known our own soul thoroughly (Julian of Norwich [1966] 1976, 161).

Similarly, John Calvin (1509-1564), pre-eminent among Reformed theologians, pointed out in his *Institutes on the Christian Religion* that

> our wisdom . . . consists almost entirely of two parts: the knowledge of God and of ourselves. But as these are connected together by many ties, it is not easy to determine which of the two precedes, and gives birth to, the other (Calvin 1962, 37).

Both Julian and Calvin hold together themselves and God in an intimate, immediate, and necessary way. Although Julian emphasizes the substance of sensuality in the soul in contrast to Calvin's more abstract knowledge of ourselves, neither splits spirit and matter. Nor do they reduce the Creator to creation. Rather, they affirm that the way we are made reflects the way God is -- we, that is humanity as humanity, are created in "the image and likeness of God."

In philosophical language, the conviction means that whatever makes up our being constitutes the Being of Being Itself. Even though the ultimate reality of the universe "transcends everything finite," that absolute reality is "the creative ground of everything finite." As Tillich put the issue of the nature of the really real, ultimate reality "is beyond what can be grasped by senses or words or thought, and it is at the same time the creative ground present in everything" (Tillich 1987, 227).

Along with Julian's substantial soul, Calvin's wisdom of ourselves, Tillich's creative ground of everything that is, and the mighty cloud of believers through the centuries, I believe there is a relation between the universe that is our brain, the universe in which we live, the way we are made, and the way life matters. I want to show how the brain can be used as a primary instrument in understanding not only how we perceive ourselves but even more how we perceive God and participate with God in our life in this world.

I am holding together religious intuition and empirical evidence in hopes of making the depths of our being more accessible to the destiny we seek. To that purpose I identify mechanisms of meaning -- the processes by which we believe and with which we believe. We are created from the dust of the earth -- the biochemical processes at the core of our environment -- and we find our affinity with the breath of life -- the transformative processes at the heart of our world.

So I ask the question of meaning differently than do the classical traditions, namely: how do we integrate -- in both our personal lives and our life together -- the dust of our brain and the breath of our mind?

Different Stories/Different Processes

The two creation narratives are well-known and have been meticulously studied (Genesis 1-2:4a; 2:4b-3:24; Anderson 1967). I propose to re-enter them in order to explain -- or suggest -- how each defined reality and to identify where and why the differences in emphases occurred in terms of the brain. Subsequent developments of how people believe build upon these two foundations. In understanding them we may begin to understand dominant patterns of belief and significant variations.

Two Narratives of Creation (RSV)

Genesis 2-3	Genesis 1
In the day that Yahweh made the earth and the heavens	When God began to create the heavens and the earth

. . .

And every living thing

then Yahweh formed Adam
of dust from the ground,
and breathed into his nostrils
the breath of life; and
Adam became a living being.
And Yahweh planted
a garden; and there put
Adam. And made to grow all
that is pleasant to the sight and
good for food, the tree of life
and the tree of the knowledge
of good and evil.
Then Yahweh said, "It
is not good for Adam to be alone;
I will make him a companion."
And Yahweh brought Adam
to see all creatures and
whatever Adam called them
that was its name.

. . .

The eyes of both were opened,
and they knew they were naked.
And they hid themselves
from the presence of Yahweh.
"Where are you hiding?"
And Adam said, "I heard the
sound of thee in the garden,
and I was afraid, because
I was naked; and I hid myself.

. . .

Yahweh drove them out
of the garden to till the ground
from which they were taken.

. . .

And God said: "Let there be
all -- everything living"
And God saw that all was good.
Then God said, "Let us make
male and female after our
  likeness." So God created
male and female in the image
and likeness of God."

And God blessed them,
"Be fruitful, fill the earth
and have dominion over it."

> God rested . . .
> These are the generations
> of the heavens and the earth
> when they were created.

In terms of the way the brain works how might we account for these contrasting stories of the context in which humanity finds itself? Each begins with a Power not our own -- we are not our own maker; yet each interprets our place in the universe in quite a different way.

A Disrupted Reality -- Genesis Two

In the first account (Genesis 2-3) God entrusts us with responsibility for the created world -- we name every "thing" that is; we test the validity of all that is taken as reality; we make what matters ultimately matter in the here-and-now. That is what life is about.

Then suddenly we experience a disrupted reality -- anxious, accountable, alienated. We hide from reality -- Yahweh God in our guts -- by basic reactions of control (attacking or withdrawing), or closeness (conniving or placating), or hesitancy (constricting or waiting). We use these strategies to avoid the truth of the situations in which we find ourselves (Ashbrook 1986).

How did that disruption come about? What are its consequences? What are we to do?

In naming the world we are creating the world. We live in that world in a mutually responsible way. In becoming aware of ourselves -- the experience of self consciousness -- we act in ways to avoid reality. To declare what life is about, then, is to insist on the imperative of right relationships and real responsibility. Belief consists of proclaiming the good news of redemption -- the setting right that which we have disrupted. In naming the world we are saving the world.

This world-transforming pattern of the left brain involves item-by-item and step-by-step processes, as these have been discovered in brain research. It is accompanied by rational-vigilant mental representational activity, as identified in cognitive research. Further, in the preference of proclamation, the pattern makes quite specific what people regard as urgently right. The vigilance of the sympathetic nervous system, harmoniously balanced with the parasympathetic system according to the perceived needs of the moment, arouses the believer to what is dangerous, as well as to what is interesting (Nathan 1976, 206-209).

To give preference to left brain activity is to recognize the active nature of the organism which we are. While we "are created" -- whether we couch that in the language of God or the language of DNA and the genetic code -- we are, nevertheless, "creators and actors" on the evolutionary stage and in the historical drama. The belief trajectory of proclamation points to God as its source of authority, yet paradoxically, the consequence points to ourselves as the instrument or locus of that authority. The mechanisms which produce the pattern of saving the world reflect the processes which are associated with the left brain.

We find that paradox embedded in the theological perspective implicit in these biblical stories of creation and their order in the canon (Anderson 1986). By theological perspective, I refer to the way in which tradition ordered the material for subsequent generations to read. The historical order of their origin is reversed in the theological perspective. Although written later, Genesis One appears first, and Genesis Two comes second, although written first.

The second story (Genesis 2-3) took shape in the ninth or tenth centuries, during the time of the United Kingdom (Vawter 1977, 17; Cross 1973, 293), so it is actually the earlier explanation. It begins with the declaration: "In the day that the Lord God made the earth and the heavens . . ." (Genesis 2:4b RSV). Note the sequence -- "*earth* and heaven." It first anchors reality on "earth," in history, with humanity at the center, and only then does it turn to reality in "heaven."

While the language of the Yahwist is mythical and imaginative -- reflective of right brain dominance -- the story itself is one of logic and analysis, which reflect left brain dominance. We find cause-and-effect, one step-at-a-time progression, and *human account-ability*. To the Yahwist writer, society had become so caught up in an uncritical espousing of its "divinely ordained" success in the monarchy that it no longer could distinguish between the sin of society and the righteousness of God. Paradoxically, the anthropocentric story of God in the Garden correlates with proclamation and left brain process. "Where are you hiding?" declares the Almighty One to humanity in its semi-autonomy.

If Yahweh is all-knowing, why the question of "where are you hiding?" Here is an expression of projection -- putting out onto others the self-consciousness that is in oneself. Experiencing the guilt of failed accountability, Adam hears that self-conscious awarenss calling him to a renewed relationship by the Creator of the context itself. An awareness of guilt/responsibility reflects a relatedness to that which is more than ourselves. Our new brain bears the relational responsiveness and responsibility for all that is around us and within us. Because we are not our own creator we are ever beholden to that which gives us life.

The narrative of suddenly hearing Yahweh God in the Garden and hiding from that judging presence reflects both an inner experience and an interpersonal reality. Conscience emerges from an identification with others -- primarily nurturing others -- mother and father. Because they have cared for us we care about what they expect of us.

Without such connectedness there is little or no conscience. We simply do not internalize the values of those around us. In the more formal language of psychopathology we become "anti-social" or "socio-pathic."

In more ordinary give-and-take, when we find ourselves up against threats to our sense of self-esteem, we react defensively. The anxiety of being confronted with that which threatens our survival as a self -- "I heard thee and hid" -- triggers in us basic survival behaviors (Ashbrook 1986). Because some people have experienced hurt in intimate relationships, under stress they look to themselves and so try to control situations in an effort to reduce their feeling of vulnerability. Because other people have experienced support in intimate relationships, under stress they look to others and so try to draw close in an effort to reduce their feeling of deficiency. And because still others have experienced a web of interrelatedness in their world, under stress they hesitate to act until they can include everyone in an effort to reduce their feeling of uncertainty.

Each of these survival reactions -- control, contact, inclusion -- serves to keep us from dealing with the responsibility of the reality of the situation. We avoid the task by defending ourselves against what we need to do. The flow of adrenalin -- the rapid heartbeat, the sudden sweat, the dry mouth, the shallow breathing -- all signal the state of emergency in which our sense of survival is at stake. In the limbic system, it is the amygdala which surges up to take over from a relaxed relationship with the environment in order to keep us alive.

The result is an intentional and deliberate balance of belief and behavior. We are called to transform the world by caring for the world as Yahweh God cares for it and for us. Moses put the issue to Israel as it is put to all of us:

> I call heaven and earth to witness against you today: I set before you life or death, blessing or curse. Choose life, then, so that you and your descendents may live, in the love of Yahweh your God, obeying Yahweh's voice, clinging to Yahweh; for in this your life consists, and on this depends your long stay in the land . . . (Deuteronomy 30:19-20 JB).

The Gospel of Mark opens with a similar expression of active intention about what matters most in our lives:

> After John had been arrested, Jesus went into Galilee. There he proclaimed the Good News from God. "The time has come," he said, "and the kingdom of God is close at hand. Repent, and believe the Good News" (Mark 1:14-15 JB).

Believers are to be doers of the Word as a result of having heard the Word. The left brain not only explains what it observes but takes initiative in being responsible for what it knows. It is vigilant -- watching over that which is needed for survival.

A Supportive Reality -- Genesis One

Now consider how reality was defined -- narrated -- in the other account. This belief reflects the way a right brain dominance would work. In this pattern we are immersed in a supportive universe; we envision the value of all that is really real; we celebrate what matters ultimately in the reality that is really here. God holds us in a gracious context -- "underneath are the everlasting arms" (Deuteronomy 3:27). That is what life is about.

There is no disruption, only smooth and steady development and differentiation -- affirmation and connectedness. We disclose reality -- the Lord God in our lives -- by basic responses of being the individual parts that we are (individuating), being a part of the whole (identifying with that which is more than we are), and weaving everything together (including everything and everyone) in expressing the goodness of life as we find it.

How did that connectedness come about? What are its consequences? How do we continue it?

In describing the world, we are affirming the world. In identifying the parts as part of the whole, we create reality. To show forth what life is about, then, is to celebrate the indicative of real relatedness and appropriate responsibility. Belief consists of manifesting the good news of creation -- the showing forth of the supportive cosmos.

This world-affirming pattern of the right brain involves processes which are all-at-once and by leaps of imagination, as these have been identified in brain research. The pattern is characterized by relational-responsive mental representations, as these have been found in cognitive research. Furthermore, in the preference of manifestation the pattern makes quite apparent what is regarded as ultimately real. The receptiveness of the parasympathetic nervous system, harmoniously balanced with the sympathetic system according to the perceived needs of the moment, enables the believer to go with the flow (Nathan 1969, 209), let go of self-preservation and allow merging with the environment for the sake of continuity and new possibilities.

To give preference to right brain activity is to recognize the receptive nature of the organism which we are. While we are intentional and responsible -- whether we couch that in the language of theology or sociology -- we are, nevertheless, creatures and parts of an evolutionary ecological system which necessitates our adapting to what it requires (Burhoe 1981). The belief trajectory of manifestation points to ourselves as the center of the universe, yet paradoxically points to God as the instrument or locus of that context in which we exist.

The right brain has taken the lead over the left in a leap of imagination and an all-at-once process. It images -- creates -- a context of wonder, of beauty, of awe, of relatedness. Although second day follows first day -- until the seventh -- and earth follows firmament even as male and female follow living creatures, the left brain sequence of cause-and-effect and of good-and-evil are more apparent than actual. As with every emotionally meaningful pattern, the pattern -- belief if you will -- appears as a result of the right brain's imaging the limbic process of: (1) deciding whether an "event" is desirable or undesirable, and then (2) determining to incorporate the meaning of that event into the ongoing reality of the person.

The basic response is the continuity and valuing of all that is. These responses serve to keep us interacting with the reality in which we find ourselves -- especially with the necessity of our relatedness with one another. In contrast to left brain-amygdala anxiousness, right brain-septal relaxed excitement flows through our body. We are alert without being aroused; eager without being frantic; caring without grasping; connected without possessing. In the limbic system, it is the septum which quickens a relaxed relationship with the environment to keep all life going.

We find that paradox of right brain dominance, as I indicated above, in the theological perspective implicit in the way the canon preserved the tradition (Anderson 1986). The later account of creation is put first, while the earlier account comes second. Note that both accounts are "explanations," conceptual formulations, interpretations of primary experience. As such, both could only come with the fuller development of the cerebral cortex as we find it in *homo sapiens.* The left hemisphere laterality, in which abstract symbolic capacity appears, is the mechanism of the meaning-making. It is associated inevitability with human consciousness. Brain researcher Michael Gazzaniga refers to it as the "interpreter," that which is "responsible for the generation of human beliefs" (Gazzaniga 1985, 5; 1988).

The first story (Genesis 1) arose during the crisis of the Babylonian captivity in the sixth century B.C.E. (Cross 1973, 324), so it actually is the later explanation. It begins with the declaration: "When God began to create the heavens and the earth . . ." (Genesis 1:1 RSV). Note the reversed sequence from the second story -- *"heavens and earth."* It orients reality in "the heavens," in the universe, without humanity, and only then does it turn to the reality of "earth."

While the language of the Priestly writer is more abstract, theological, and therefore left brain than the concrete imagery of the second account, the story itself is one of an imaginative wholeness. In contrast to the competitive struggle between order (Marduk) and chaos (Tiamat), as ennuciated in Babylon's great national epic, *Enuma elish* (Pritchard 1969, 60-72) -- a primordial conflict between two halves of the universe -- we find an all-at-once, leap of imagination, making-whole in which the many facets of life show forth *the blessedness of divine unity*. Our attention is directed to the appearance of things instead of to their underlying functions (cf. Levy and Trevarthen 1976).

In this first account of creation, nothing is depreciated or segregated as in the second account. There is no forbidden tree; no tragic fall; no alienating anxiety. While creation is never the greatest good, it is ever the very good (Genesis 1:31). Even the terrifying monsters of the deep (Genesis 1:21) are called good. The natural order may feel chaotic, yet for the believer, the liberated ones, order is neither cancelled nor rejected. From the experience of the Exodus, Israel looked back to the creation and confessed that "the God who was active at the beginning of her history was likewise active at the beginning of the world's history" (Anderson 1967, 38).

The Priestly writer did not address the despair of the exiles with an analysis of the competing gods of light and dark. Rather, the writer lifted up a vision of the sun and the moon and the stars as placed in the sky by One Creator, One Reality which is a Relational Reality. No tyrannical Marduk subdued a chaotic Tiamat. Instead, all monsters of the deep lived together because they originated from one origin. Everything is located and differentiated in a contextual universe -- day and night, water and land, vegetation and creatures, life and human life. There is no need to control the cosmos and its creatures through ritual. "God completed the work. . . . Such were the origins of heaven and earth when they were created" (Genesis 2:1-4a). The passage witnesses to the relatedness of everything in all creation, including humanity.

The result is an intouch and spontaneous (non-self-conscious) integrating of believing and behaving. We experience pleasure and contentment, excitement and support. In contrast to the rational cosmos conceived of by the Greeks, biblical faith perceives Yahweh as personally and intimately involved with creation. Within that divinely "voiced" order -- in the beginning was the Word (Genesis 1:1 and John 1:1) -- each creature is made to fulfill the intended will of its Creator (Anderson 1962a). Each particle proclaims its promises of glory. Believers manifest the enlivening presence of Holy Presence itself. The right brain takes the lead over the left in responding to the meaning-ful context in which it finds itself (based on its incorporating that meaning through the imagery it generates).

The differences in left and right brain processes help make these two narratives of the context in which we find ourselves sensible. In addition to historical and literary analyses, cognitive styles and preferences suggest how the contrasts could occur. Further, distinguishing the cognitive styles enables us to understand more fully the various ways in which people create their systems of belief about the way things are and how we are to live in terms of that reality.

Basic Plots

Consider again our triune brain -- the primal mind of instinctual behavior, the mammalian mind of emotional behavior, and the new mind of rational behavior. Paul MacLean, who identified these three levels of organization, suggests that we can think of these minds in terms of literature, namely, that there appears to be "an irreducible number of basic plots and associated emotions":

> In metaphorical terms, we might imagine that the reptilian brain provides the basic plots and actions in our lives, that the limbic brain emotionally influences the

development of these plots; and that, finally, the non-mammalian brain has the capacity to elaborate upon the basic plots and emotions in as many ways as there are authors (MacLean 1977, 159-160).

That metaphorical analogy of MacLean identifies the finiteness and freedom of our life.

In our reptilian mind we live through our senses. Think of it as our brain when we are babies. In later years we use it to relive the fears of our earliest ancestors -- the fear of the dark (unknown), the fear of falling, the fear of being separated from that which gives security, the fear of not having a place.

In our mammalian mind we live through our emotions. Think of it as our brain when our environment is "hot" and so calls for our deciding whether it is pleasurable and desirable or painful and undesirable. We hear "loud" and give it an image of blasting; we image "mothering" and give it a feeling (usually) of closeness.

In our new mind we live through our thinking. Think of it as our brain when we are shaping the landscape. Everything is catalogued -- first through the senses, then with emotions, and finally through words. We take a piece of wood or stone and make a statue; we combine chemical elements to alter our moods; we create instruments to extend the range of our senses. Most of all, we imagine "the way things are" and behave accordingly.

Although there seem to be only a limited number of scenerios of what it means to be human, we interpret these basic plots in an infinite number of ways -- variations on the theme of being the human beings that we are. We vary the ways we preserve our sense of self, even as we vary the ways we preserve community and continue our species. In religious language, Tillich called that the courage to be as oneself and the courage to be as a part of the whole (Tillich 1952). In psychological language, it is identified as concern with the self and concern with the system in which the self participates (Nichols 1987).

Concern for the self -- what at its basic level is literal survival and at its most developed level is courage to be as oneself -- arises from the activation of the sympathetic nervous system mediated through the amygdala and arousal. Literal survival tends to be limited to the physical environment; psychological and spiritual survival and courage tend to be influenced by the interpersonal world of meaning in which we place ourselves (cf. Sullivan 1953; Anchin and Kiesler 1982).

Concern for the system -- what at its basic level is the literal preservation of the species and at its most developed level is courage to be as a part of the whole -- comes with the activation of the parasympathetic nervous system mediated through the septum and relaxation. Literal continuity is now taking the form of concern for the entire ecological environment -- the atmosphere we breathe and the water and land upon which we depend; psychological and spiritual cooperation and community require the whole human family if we are to live together on this tiny speck in an infinite spaciousness.

The balance between self-and-setting, thereby, affects both how we act in the immediate moment and what we believe about the surrounding context of our universe.

Plots develop according to the emotional climate we each perceive and frame. Those developments reflect what has come to be known as the "felt-meaning" of situations (Gendlin 1962) -- the way we experience them in our body and imagine their importance with our mind. Life is seldom neutral. We construe it in terms of feeling and thought, emotion and concept, sensation and sensibility -- all integrated by means of the images we create.

For instance, a plot fired by survival vigilance unfolds differently from one nurtured by shared values. If we feel attacked, we distance ourselves from others -- either by fleeing or fighting. On the other hand, if we feel affirmed, we move closer to others -- either by helping them or being helped by them. The resulting drama becomes either one of conflict (activated by the aggressive amygdala) or one of cooperation (activated by the affiliative septum).

The new brain expands on those plots and emotions. The way we develop the plots bears the stamp of our distinct personalities and the kind of stories we tell. Our own idiosyncratic qualities are as unique in their nuances as finger prints, handwriting, walking, and talking (Williams 1956). No other story is ever quite the same as our story. In telling who we are we each narrate a unique variation on the human story itself.

What I am contending for is this: under conditions of anxiety in the mind and stress in the body (and anxiety/stress are always of a single reality), we fall back onto limited and restricting patterns of knowing, believing, belonging, and behaving (Selye 1976; Benson 1979; Borysenko 1987; Rossi 1986; Ornstein and Sobel 1988). The consequence is a runaway limbic system (Hampden-Turner 1981, 84). An appropriate balance (between survival of the self and supporting the group) has been destroyed under an emergency mentality -- what in theological terms is called an eschatological apocalypticism, a pessimistic expectation that the end of the world is at hand (Richardson and Bowden 1983, 183-186, 28-29).

Under those circumstances, the configurations of our making meaning stand out as central tendencies, regardless of time and place and people. Individual variations range between those who look to others in a histrionic/hysterical way, to those who depend only upon themselves and act against others in an autonomous or narcissistic way, to those who stay locked within an immediate situation with compulsive or obsessive interpersonal maneuvers (Horowitz [1978] 1986). Under stress -- what traditional theology has called the condition of sin -- we are more alike than different. We are thrown back upon our basic assumptions -- emotional (Colman and Bexton 1975; Colman and Geller 1985) and ideational -- about the way to survive in an uncertain world: we attach ourselves to others; we distance ourselves from others; or we include others (Ashbrook 1986).

Each of these strategies is dysfunctional in that each allows us to avoid the work of reality -- whether by closeness to, control of, or connectedness with others. By acting on the fantasy assumption we make, we fail to take responsibility necessary to engage reality. In the language of the creation narrative of the Garden, we hide from Yahweh God (Genesis 3:8-13). We distort what is real, we deny what is right, we destroy what is meant to be, namely, shared life, in human community, within a universe of influences that supports life as we know it. At least, that is the proposition I am advancing.

Similar Plots

Much that I am identifying with the way the brain works has been observed and reflected upon through the centuries. We have known about analytic and holistic contrasts, about survival of the self and preservation of community. There is little which is basically new (Ashbrook 1984c, 5-9; Bakan 1966; Springer and Deutsch [1981] 1985, 236-239).

For instance, in her classic description of mysticism, Evelyn Underhill (1961, 346) characterized two different approaches to the divine: the ascetic -- or abstract -- way as represented by a trip to the Antarctica and the joyful -- or immediate -- way as symbolized by a wedding feast.

Other instances include Hannah Arendt's analysis of "The Life of the Mind." She examined the two-world theory in the old metaphysical dichotomy between (true) Being and (mere) Appearance (Arendt [1971, 1977] 1978, 23-30). Or, in moving toward "an integrated cognitive science," Gardner (1985) explored the many variations of such contrasts as molar/molecular, top-down/bottom-up, central processing/peripheral processing, description/depictive, and vertical truth/horizontal impressions.

Why bother talking about the brain with all of this understanding from the past? This is the question raised by some critics. Specialized information about the brain only duplicates the accrued wisdom of the ages, so they contend.

Centuries of experience have sifted and crystallized basic scenerios of human orientation, organization, and action. Current research is identifying more specifically "how" we function as we do and "why." The presence of difference, of variation, of diversity, of pluralism -- call it what we will -- discloses fundamental brain activity, even "biochemical individuality," as one scientist labelled it (Williams 1956).

But what previous generations have learned through the wisdom of lived experience is now available as specific information. The fact that we now know about ourselves and our universe with more precision only heightens the wondrous mystery of how we are put together. Discernible regularities are not the same as controllable processes. Our mastery of knowledge will never result in our mastery of the mystery that is our universe.

We live in a context not of our own making, and therefore in an environment to which we must accommodate. Within that environment we create a world, but our world must accord with the demands of those evolutionary processes or we destroy ourselves and sabotage that environment. We are very close to doing that in our time. So the issue of the meaning and means of what matters most to genuine human life takes on compelling importance. To understand belief in light of the brain offers the possibility of a more informed knowledge of "how" to live, even as to understand the brain in light of belief compels us to recognize the reality of "what it means" to live an inclusive and caring life.

In order to identify the issue between what we know about the brain and how we have believed I use one person's experience of that struggle. It is a personal response, triggered by working with the ideas of this book, and called forth by the human need to make sense of her experience.

One Person's Plot

Barbara Stinchcombe is a free-lance editor. She also works as an editorial assistant in the dissertation office at the University of Chicago as well as being a poetess in her own right. She lives and works in a sophisticated scientific world and academic community. In reading a newspaper series on brain research she voiced outrage at the following assertion by Richard Masland, a neuroscientist at Harvard University and Massachusetts General Hosptial in Boston:

> Down the road we're going to be able to make any kind of person we want using molecular biology. . . . We're going to be able to create from birth a person who is tall, has blue eyes and an IQ of 400. The technology is going to happen to do that. The people who are going to develop those techniques are going to do it in order to cure mental diseases and other disorders. But once they've learned how to do it, the Pandora's box will be opened (Kotulak 1988).

Stinchcombe criticized the lack of struggle in this vision of the future -- the absence of moral character, the mechanizing of human beings. The attitude is "the atom bomb all over again," implying the mastery of physical power without the monitoring mystery of human accountability. What is missing, she concluded, is "an ideal [image] which we serve."

My effort to hold together the brain and belief elicited from her the following understanding of the basic story plot of her life. With her permission I share it as illustrative of the process of uniting what people "know" of life from inside their experienced world and what we are "learning about" life from observation of that experience.

Sensations

> My understanding of how my brain functions [involves]
> how it has -- from [its] first forming in my body -- in-
> formed me about the world to which my body was
> formed. At first my knowledge was through my senses,
> but even in that instance, the senses carried information
> to the brain. I learned "hot" by sensation. "Mother" by
> sensation.

Stinchcombe is pointing toward the basic genetic code carried in
the chromosomal make-up of every living creature. Because of
that code our body "knows how" to respond to the world within itself -- like breathing, heart rate, temperature level, and maintaining the equilibrium of its internal milieu -- as well as how to begin
to relate to the world around.

The genetic code rarely functions by itself. Not only is the body
linked with the culture code, the accumulated wisdom of how
people become people and belong to the group, but the body is inevitably under the active shaping of the world by the neocortex.
Because so much of the brain, especially the neocortex, is not
wired for prescribed instinctual behaviors, the brain learns how we
are to get along in the world. And we learn that by our interaction
with others. It is this culture code process which Stinchcombe has
identified with such initial sensations as "hot" and "mother" and
which associations she next ties to language.

> Later words were put to the information the senses car-
> ried. With age the importance of the senses regressed
> as the importance of language superseded them. The
> mind made a jump carrying itself and the person it em-
> bodied [namely me] into "civilized" society, a world in
> which people communicated with words and gestures;
> my senses becoming sometimes those very things I had
> to learn to control following the subscribed patterns of
> behavior of the society in which I lived.

She has described the transition from a sensory-motor reality to a speech-oriented world. In terms of the functioning brain it is a transition from the older levels of the reptilian instincts and the mammalian emotions to the new level of conscious structuring and strategizing by means of the left and right hemispheres. A growing awareness of limits and permission -- "No's" and "Yes's" -- increasingly characterized her life -- what developmental researchers describe as a transition from the initial stage of trust vs. mistrust to the learning of control in the stage of autonomy vs. shame and doubt.

Conflict Between Good and Evil

Sensations were no longer simply pleasurable or painful, to be explored or to be avoided. Now the sensations of pleasure or pain were defined by messages coming from the powerful people around her, particularly mother and father. The world began to lose its "wholeness" as it more and more took on the image of contrast -- positive and negative, good and bad, the good-me and the not-me with the bad-me in between.

> The potential for good and evil existed alongside me. Some good things were learned, some taught -- the intent being to form me into an acceptable member of my society. Gradually some good things happened because I willed them to happen by acting them out. These were actions that primarily carried their good within themselves -- good for the sake of good? -- or because the action or will to action came from inside me and related to another person's good by making them happy? So the idea of another kind of good grew in my mind.

> On the other side existed the idea of evil -- to do bad things. Again, as with the things I learned or was taught about being good, I was similarly taught regarding evil. By acting out certain bad things I would risk becoming a bad and unacceptable member of society. Just as there was another kind of good beyond those things learned

and taught, there was another kind of evil beyond -- an evil that could harm me inside.

Instinctual responses and intentional awareness were experienced as two separate spheres of motivation. The old cortex and the new cortex are differentiated in their functioning -- so separate as to result in St. Paul's not understanding how it was that he did not do what he wanted, but instead he did the very thing he hated (Romans 7:15). Similarly, the way Stinchcombe behaved could conflict with what she thought. The world assumed more of an interpersonal milieu and less of simply a physical reality. What others expected had to be taken into account as well as what she found inside herself.

Internalizing Values

In terms of moral development theory she was beginning to internalize the values of her parents and society. She was moving from a stage of conformity towards an individualized conscience -- not simply do what the authorities say because they say it, but do what the authorities have said because it helps me feel more comfortable with myself. She was sensing a convergence between outer demand and inner necessity.

The apparent split between good and evil moved from an external arena to a more internal experiencing of conflicting values. If the tension seemed to have originated outside of herself and had its source in others, now the tension arose inside herself and in the personal world which she was creating. Even more surprising to her, she began to discover that what was being handed on to her from the past -- values, beliefs, morals as coded in culture and especially religious history -- involved a subtle and complicated convergence of how she acted, how she felt, and how the universe was actually ordered.

Slowly I discovered these evil things that could harm me on the inside were already embodied in the moral code as given to Moses. A connection was being made --

slowly -- between [1] acting out good and evil; [2] how it
felt inside; and [3] how that interior feeling was related
to God through the commandments.

This discovery was not made as clearly as I am relating it
here, but obliquely. It was part of my early religious
training -- the exercise of (or acting out of) good and
evil being part of it -- and the existence of those two (2)
forces, when they engaged in conflict with my inner
being, brought about feelings inside me that were
generated from inside -- a force different from the force
society used in teaching me about good and bad so as to
become an acceptable human being.

From what we know about the brain, Stinchcombe was experiencing the three minds of her one brain: namely, the instinctual mind
of how she behaved; the emotional mind which held together
pleasure and pain, self and others, the past and the present; and
the conscious mind which made sense of the many facets of inner
and outer experience by interpreting what was and planning what
might be.

At the lowest level these [two forces of good and evil]
were sensations or feelings -- used in the same manner
as my exterior senses informed my brain about the
world in infancy. But the sensing now was interior and
thus somewhat different. Much later in life I made a
connection between these interior sensations and the
moral laws I had been taught.

It is impossible to know how a religious sense would
have developed without it having been taught by my
parents and church. The question is [whether] the
beginning sensations of good and evil and the notion I
could act [these feelings] out have been enough to have
brought me to a force I understood as God? I do not
know.

Stinchcombe identifies the crucial interface between facts and faith. Are sensations the source of spiritual reality? Is awareness of something being "good or bad" -- and the capacity to act in either a "good or bad" way -- the origin of a consciousness of an ever-present, all-knowing, ever-demanding God?

She voices doubt about whether the inner experience between something "good" and something "bad" was sufficient in itself to bring her to the realization of "a force" she understood "as God."

> At bottom I believe faith is something learned over time. And this is how it happened for me. I came to believe in God because I was taught to believe in God -- that I ought to believe in God. So I believed as expected of me as a child. God was a powerful force. Sometimes I responded to this great unknown with the usual challenge children use -- "If you're so powerful strike me dead." As I challenged [God or that unknown force] for signs, sometimes I also truly believed from fear of what would happen if I did not.

Doubts and beliefs reflect the maturing of the two hemispheres. There emerges a dialectical distance between sensations within the body and ideas within the head, between what we sense viscerally and what we are able to say verbally, between how we actually act and what we feel we "should" do. We experience ourselves moving back and forth between what we observe -- including our inner feelings -- and how we interpret what those observations mean. We find ourselves inevitably working to "make sense" of our world. The left brain is always putting what it observes into a coherent rationale to explain "what is."

The sensible interpretation -- belief -- comes initially from others. Parents, family, friends, teachers, ministers all tell us what to think and why things are the way they are. Part of that "telling" of "the truth" includes reference to an all-powering yet unseen presence which people call "God."

At the emotional level of survival, the message comes across as "God will getcha if you aren't good," which translates into our doing what the authority says we should do. The conscious mind takes the point of view of the powerful other. However, in the very act of taking over the view point of others we begin to reflect upon that viewpoint, to wonder about it, to question it, to find ourselves rejecting it for a viewpoint of our own making or to agree with it in terms of our own logic.

Questioning and Consciousness

Questioning carries the seeds of its own uncertainty. We cannot "not" question questioning. The rational mind never loses its origin in the emotional and instinctual minds. The rational mind, as we are learning, interprets what is happening as desirable or undesirable, based on a decision in the limbic system. Based on that decision we act according to the rationale we provide. We act in a way that integrates survival of the self, continuity of the species, and care for those who are vulnerable (particularly infants). Some part of us -- most likely the inhibiting activity of the left brain fed by the affiliating activity of the right brain -- fears that if we do not act in ways that take others into account something undesirable will happen to us.

> Now as a grown, believing adult, I occasionally have a sense of awe at this power which created the universe, and it is at such times I remember the Psalm: "What is man that Thou should care for him" [Psalm 8:4]? And there is still a trace of childish fear that makes me wonder whether we really know what we are asking of God. What if God did exercise His power in response to our requests and petitions?

The residue of a child's strange mixture of a sense of omnipotence and a sense of entitlement to be taken care of never completely disappears. If we want something, we deserve to get it. If we ask for something, it is ours for the asking. We have no obligation or responsibility other than to voice the impulses of our hearts. Ask

God to do for us what we regard as necessary for our own life. So runs the logic of childish emotion.

Yet that emotional childishness is mediated through an objectifying consciousness of ourselves and of the universe in which we live. What we ask and how we act somehow go together *in us* and not simply in an external world.

> God answers our requests and petitions through us when we exercise our will to goodness on those occasions when we act more in God's image. I am glad it works that way, for when I do good things that reflect this image, I feel closer to God. It's a quiet, loving, communal feeling that I can appreciate as an adult, but also sense as a child in relation to a wise and understanding parent. Thus the feeling also carries a sense of security.

As a person conscious of herself and her experience, aware of a world around her and a universe in which she is but a part, Stinchcombe voices the coming together -- in her articulated consciousness -- of the bodily reality of the primal and emotional minds with the imaginative and interpretive reality of the rational mind. The autonomic nervous system balances a relaxation which allows her to be a part of a larger whole and an alertness which knows that "what is good for all" is "what is good for self." An openness or vulnerability becomes a childlike innocence or a trusting of the forces working inside her as reflecting the forces she engages in the world around her.

Making It On Her Own

At this point in life Stinchcombe began to experience and express her own initiative and her own capacity to think things through. She could act on her own conscious choices in ways which might differ significantly from others. She did not feel dependent upon others or beholden to them.

So, I learned from my parents and church to believe in God. As I grew older and practised in the use of thought and thinking things out, I left their teaching and belief -- I was too old for it; it was a lot of superstition; and how could miracles happen as related in some Holy Book? Reality was life -- my breathing in and out -- reality was what people created with their minds working to create machines and medicines to improve life now; to save people from illness.

It wasn't some mythical God doing these things, but man [sic] in the potential he had in his smartness and ingenuity. God didn't invent machines. Man did. At best, if God was embodied in nature -- His universe -- then His acting through nature was totally cruel. And that man wanted to use his force to control this wild, evil force made total sense to me.

At one point learning that in the theological community they were announcing "God is dead," I concluded at last those people are getting in touch with reality. Then I wondered what they would do vis-a-vis their teaching. Perhaps they'd have to close down. It sounded kind of a sad thing. But right on time, right on line.

She is expressing an awareness of tragedy, absurdity, and cruelty which pervade so much of life. No right thinking person would construct and continue such a questionable habitat. She felt sympathy for those whose life and livelihood depended upon a dead deity.

At the same time real life did not involve or require God. In fact, those who thought and talked in terms of God were inept, inadequate, less than intelligent. "Brains" was where things counted -- the academic, the scientific, the knowable.

I grew older. Lived in a community of academicians who with every confidence asserted the center of the universe was man [sic]. There was always a feeling of strength, thought, figuring out, finding answers. Our world did not have to be an unknown and superstitious place. Look at how smart we were -- without God. I often made fun of believers, and regularly swore using God's name -- He was so much disregarded, fallen out of use in my mind.

I received a come-uppance once. While conversing with a neighbor and swearing in my usual manner using God's name, my neighbor, a quiet, retiring type of person said, "You know, I'm a believer -- a Christian -- and when you talk that way, it offends me."

Her statement startled me. I acknowledged her feeling offended and did not quite manage an apology except to nod. But clearly I remembered the exchange. And it did make me more circumspect. Christians after all were people too with feelings.

More To Life Than Mastery

Like a sturdy shrub, Stinchcombe continued to grow, to send the roots of her reality deeper into the soil of her own reality and outward into the atmosphere of others' reality. Like so many of us, in growing older she discovered that she was not as smart as she had thought. There was more to life than she could manage.

I grew older. My father died. Slowly I started to think about the mystery which was his person. And time after time I came back to a picture of him as a person who just totally had thrown his person in the trust of God. It didn't make sense to me. But the simpleness of his faith always left a feeling of curiosity. Clearly I couldn't separate him from his belief in trying to understand who he was -- the good things in his person always led back to this belief in God.

At the same time the gods in the society in which I lived were turning out to be sometimes quite insubstantial people with no more final answers than the God I had renounced. Yet life went on -- full of enough problems to occupy my time and thought. But not so [completely] occupied: the mind also considered, as is its custom, who is the person I am?

Midlife experiences bring with them encounters with death, with the finiteness of what matters to us as well as with the preciousness of life together.

The dominant left brain no longer rules supreme. It takes note of the more subtle purposes and promises in our relationships with each other and with life itself. The interpretive left brain searches beyond the surface explanation of a shovel being associated with a chicken -- as in the experiment with Paul -- to discerning other sources of information, information from the right hemisphere and from the older strata of the brain.

Soon our conscious mind reflects upon its own reflection, aware that it is not the source of its existence nor the final arbiter of its understanding. The new brain realizes it is a part of something other than its own self-conscious consciousness. Our sense of self emerges from a context vaster than anything we can fully grasp or even imagine.

Stinchcombe continues her reflection on her own personhood and the part the brain and mind play in that reality. Moreover, despite her wondering about questioning scientific mastery and the self in control of its self, she thought of faith -- its emotional source -- and belief -- its conceptualization -- as having functional value for less than adequate individuals. But faith and belief had no substantive value or reality in the basic scheme of things.

In periods of such reflection two (2) sets of images and ideas were reviewed for comparison: [1] the world in which I lived -- scholarly and scientifically oriented; and

[2] the world of faith in which my father had existed and people such as my neighbor who had said she was offended when she listened to me swear using God's name.

Willy-nilly, I came back to considering God again. I changed my swear words. I observed people in the world (outside my close and closed community) -- how they lived -- specifically how many lived in extremely trying circumstances and were held fast by a faith in God. Or I'd read stories in the paper. Slowly the idea of faith -- having faith -- became a possible force as my self-awarensss in the possibility of becoming a sympathizer of this community developed.

My reluctance was often permeated by the memory of a friend who had turned Christian and how, though we tried to understand her decision intellectually, we could not. We could only understand it in terms of her psychological needs. If believing in God held her world together and helped her sanity, who were we to fault it?

Nevertheless, it was peculiar because she had fallen away from our faith -- the faith where we were as people in the very center of a universe which we could create in our image. Why wasn't that enough for her? Because that limited faith wasn't adequate served to prove: 1) the depth of her emotional problems, and 2) the need of something mythical and unworldly.

Because of her choice, even in need, she was regarded [by us] as less than "intellectual." We felt ashamed for her; sorry she was that way. We argued against her, but nowhere did we argue with an understanding that the place or ground from which she argued was worthy of consideration. That [attitude of condescension on our part] about said it for religion and belief in God for us.

Stinchcombe reflects the limited analysis of the left brain as it tries to understand and voice the limitless experience of the right brain and below that of the older brain. We always know more than we can say and so experience ourselves saying less than we actually know. Further, we often experience ourselves saying things that do not "add up" or "make sense" even though the ideas seem reasonable in themselves.

"We Cannot Reinvent Ourselves"

It is this uncertainty about what she knows, about what she understands, about what she experiences, and about what she observes that keeps haunting Stinchcombe.

Nonetheless the mind does continue always to sort itself -- trying to resolve who is this person I am in the world in which this person I am exists. And it is difficult to understand one's presence without one's past -- these influences from the past influencing how the present person presents him or herself in the world.

We cannot reinvent ourselves -- perhaps this is what the 20th century man [sic] with blind faith in technology tried to do and failed in this respect.

Even though we live in the present and towards the future, she begins to realize our dependence upon the past -- where we have come from, the actual source of our life here-and-now. She is a genetic heritage as well as a cultural heritage, with her life in the universe as well as her life in a family. The mind, somehow, is part and parcel of both a personal world and a supportive environment. Instead of "inventing" herself or "reinventing" herself, she discovered she was coming back to herself, the deep self that expresses itself in all surface expressions.

In this newer phase of trying to understand myself I didn't try to reinvent myself but admitted into my mind images from my past -- those were images and teachings about God.   Though I, as an adult, had regarded myself philosophically as a humanitarian (that I knew good from bad, could sort them out and would not willingly hurt another person) I went back to much earlier ideas of these two (2) forces of good and evil and considered again the moral laws that God had given to Moses.

Such considerations left me puzzled for it felt as though a new territory was being opened in my mind -- there was something inside me not yet discovered.   And when finally I had returned to my faith the conclusion of this search was a simple deciding that I do believe in God.   I said it out loud so I could hear it and the emotional and thinking part of my brain must have been in accord because it felt right to believe and I cried because it also felt like coming home.

The split between the forces of good and bad or the split between feeling and thinking or the split between self-consciousness and an awareness of her own inner reality receded.   Conflict between an analytical left brain vigilance and a relational right brain responsiveness disappeared.   In its stead there emerged a single experience of integrating symbolic and subsymbolic processing, a wholeness in which she simply let go of self-conscious rationality and found she was sustained by a gracious God working through the organizing activity of her brain.

She is describing an integrated functioning brain.   The corpus callosum is exchanging information between the strategies of step-by-step and of all-at-once in a collaborative way; the limbic connection is integrating instinct and emotion even as it reincorporates the ideas and images of the neocortex into an ongoing psychic reality.   Genetic information and cultural information combine to disclose the information of the cosmos itself -- God as the ultimate reality which shapes, selects, and supports optimal adaptation in our universe.

As she puts it, "it felt as though a new territory was being opened in my mind . . . something inside me not yet discovered." And when she let go of the control exercised by consciousness and self-consciousness, she found "a simple" inner choice, deeper than words yet capable of a word, namely, "I do believe in God. I said it out loud so I could hear it and the emotional and thinking part of my brain must have been in accord because it felt right . . . like coming home." No wonder she cried -- with joy.

"Coming Home"

In realizing that we cannot reinvent ourselves she experienced "coming home." That metaphor quickens our longing to be "at home" in the universe. It links the conceptual understanding of the neocortex with the older brain. The two hemispheres of the conscious mind find their source in the older emotional and primal minds, and in that reconnection one experiences a congruence, a fit between what one feels, what one thinks, what one imagines, and what one says. The metaphor helps us to let go of calculating vigilance, to relax, to allow ourselves to take in information necessary for balancing our participation in community, our care for others, our survival as ourselves as a part of the whole, and our assimilating new experience into the ongoing reality that is our own.

The felt-meaning of the way life is is that of "coming home."

> As time passed my belief filled out a part of my person, making sense of feelings and thoughts I had about life -- a philosophy developed -- a way of looking at things that keep expanding the universe for me. Throughout [the process], the more I became aware of myself in the context of a believer the more I became aware of God, the more I became aware of life.

> Every believer has his or her own personal testimony of belief. I talk about mine at this point because I am putting it alongside what I understand you [Ashbrook] are proposing: to use the brain to join [that reality] with [an

understanding of] God. You are trying to show how people might use their [actual brain as an object of understanding] to expand (1) their ideas of themselves, (2) their ideas of the universe, and (3) their ideas of God.

My editorial consultant experiences the difficulty of moving -- conceptually, emotionally, faith-wise -- from the literal brain to "coming home" to oneself by coming back to God. The cognitive leap from what we know about the brain to what we mean by God -- and the reality of God's reality -- is not self-evident. It does, in truth, reflect an act of faith -- a decision below consciousness, which we then translate into an articulated belief, an interpretation of what we know in our very being and what we carry in our body/brain of the universe of which we are a part.

Stinchcombe points out the easier task of linking the brain with the ideas of self and of the universe. The ecology movement, the notion of all one world, the medical/scientific research which seeks to incorporate a human being as having a mind and body that work together -- these each are intelligible connections. But the more difficult task is joining that unity of the brain-mind/genes-culture/body-universe/dust-breath to God in some plausible way.

In her own self-reflection she now recognizes an unbroken connection between the outer world and her inner reality. She voices the conviction that what she has been given through the religious heritage and through the values of her upbringing are actually the core of the way she has been made as a person. For her, religious tradition and family life are now interpreted as outward expressions of the organizing reality of her inner reality, most particularly her brain as it holds together the impersonal genetic code and the more personal socio-cultural codes.

But God? How does God fit in all of this? God has become a living reality for her -- a context of gracious meaning, but how is God known, understood, related to, and connected with the brain of three minds? While she joins her faith with others in testifying to the experience of our being "fearfully and wonderfully" made (Psalm 139:14 KJ), she asks "how" does the brain make the mind of God understandable?

In the next chapter I try to describe mechanisms of belief, the ways the brain makes the intentionality of God understandable.

CHAPTER SEVEN

MECHANISMS OF BELIEF

My parents were wandering Arameans.
They went down into Egypt . . .
The Egyptians ill-treated us . . .
We called on Yahweh . . .
who heard our voice and saw our misery . . .
and Yahweh brought us out . . .
(Deuteronomy 26:5-11 JB)

People tell stories which tell who they are and what they believe. The story in Deuteronomy 26:5-11 is told as a story of the human family. We wander through the world looking for a place to be. We settle down only to find we are done in, victimized, alienated, cut off from one another and from the resources of life and livelihood. We cry out for deliverance. And Yahweh God acts to bring us out of bondage.

The story reflects "the story of our life" as a people of "The Book." Behind every theological doctrine and every statement of faith lies a story, a tale, a narrative -- combining myth, fable and history (see Alter 1981). We voice who we are through the stories we tell (Goldberg 1981 and 1982). Such is the faith that makes for life. Yet precisely such faith sets up a dilemma. How do we live out the reality which redeems life from destruction?

Essayist E.B. White wrote about the dilemma:

> If the world were merely seductive, that would be easy.
> If it were merely challenging, that would be no problem,
> but I arise in the morning torn between a desire to im-
> prove [or save] the world and a desire to enjoy [or savor]

the world. This makes it hard to plan the day (quoted by Fox 1972, 98).

To save or to savor, to improve or to enjoy, to make changes or to let be, to be aroused or to be relaxed -- that is the dilemma confronting most people much of the time. How do we plan our day? How do we go about the task of living? What are the beliefs which shape reality? How do we live out the story of our lives?

Through the ages people have experienced life as messy, chaotic, destructive, hostile. It cried out to be changed. It needed straightening up. It simply was not what it was meant to be. At the same time, other people -- often the same people -- have experienced life as meaningful, orderly, creative, caring. It provided sustenance. It sang with joy. It surely was what it was supposed to be.

And, of course, always there have been those who have lurched between life as messy and life as meaningful, between a gracious context and a crushing context. Through the ages people have asked whether God is a loving God or is God a wrathful God? Are we meant to save the world or to savor the world?

For Christians, "storytelling is history-telling" (Goldberg 1981 and 1982, 148; Sanders 1987a). Every story is structured in a way which enables listeners to follow it and thereby take it into their own life stories (Goldberg 1981 and 1982, 173-184). The experiences and stories of life's stresses have led theologians and philosophers to emphasize two aspects of reality: saving the world, which requires world-transforming activity to straighten up the messiness, and savoring the world, which invites world-affirming activity to sustain life's meaningfulness. God as Creator of life is viewed as possessing two natures: a redeeming nature which shapes life according to what God intends life to become and a creating nature which supports what God knows life to be. These views characterize traditional ways people have believed God to be, especially in western thought (Hanson 1982; Harvey 1964, 62-64, 201-202).

In Israel's oldest confession of faith -- what is called the Historical Credo -- the story of its life -- the awareness of God's creating activity only comes after the experience of God's saving activity (von Rad [1965] 1966, 3-8; Westerman [1971] 1974, 116):

> My father [Abraham with my mother Sarah] was a wandering Aramean. He went down into Egypt . . . The Egyptians ill-treated us . . .we called on Yahweh . . .[who] heard our voice and saw our misery . . .and Yahweh brought us out . . . (Deuteronomy 26:5-11 JB).

Because they experienced liberation from slavery, the Hebrews saw God's power everywhere. Thus, they included natural forces within the plan of the One they knew as the Lord of history. Reality was of a piece, an integrated and integrating whole -- nature and history, physical reality and purposive reality.

> His wisdom made the heaven,
>   his love is everlasting! . . .
> He struck down the first-born of Egypt,
>   his love is everlasting!
> And brought Israel out,
>   his love is everlasting!
> (Psalm 136:5-12 JB)

> Thus says God, Yahweh
> he who created the heavens and spread
> them out, who gave shape to the earth
> of what came from it, who gave breath to its people and
> life to the creatures that move in it:
> "I, Yahweh, have called you to serve the cause of
> right . . ."
> (Isaiah 42:5-7 JB).

The prophets emphasized God's creative activity by insisting upon righteousness as a universal imperative (e.g., Amos 4:12). God has redeemed us, so we are to "serve the cause of right." So the story went and so the story was meant to be.

People experienced the liberating God as a loving God. They no longer separated God's redeeming activity from God's creating activity. God was God -- One, Whole, Integrated, Inclusive. Second Isaiah affirms that deeper unity:

...thus says Yahweh,
who created you, Jacob,
who formed you, Israel:
Do not be afraid,
for I have redeemed you
(Isaiah 43:1ff JB).

The Reality that brought order out of chaos is the same Reality that pushed back the waters of the Red Sea in leading Israel out of bondage (Isaiah 51:9-10). Because of their deliverance, that motley band of nomads saw God at work on behalf of humanity throughout the whole universe (Goldberg 1981 and 1982, 153, 216-225). We are made, they declared, for making reality meaningful.

Through the centuries believers have described such experience in many ways. The Christian faith affirms: "In the beginning was the Word . . . And the Word became flesh and dwelt among us . . . we have beheld [God's] glory" (John 1:1, 14 RSV). Simply to lift up "The Word" or Logos as the ordering and orderly structuring of the universe obscures different ways in which Christians have used the concept.

Those in the tradition of church theologian Karl Barth have emphasized The Word as incarnation, the Word as biblical text, and The Word as proclamation. In contrast, those in the tradition of philosophical theologian Paul Tillich have pointed to The Word as I have just suggested, namely, as the logos within the life of God, the logos uttered in creation, and the prophetic Word "manifest in the history of revelation." Neither orientation, however, could deny the other forms. Each expresses a different facet of the divine presence in human life (Price 1986). Within these various expressions lies the reality of people giving voice to their experiences in terms of meaning-making and story telling (Alter 1981; Goldberg 1981 and 1982).

Words are transformations of the deep structure of meaning-making. In putting the issue that way I am drawing upon two distinct domains of discourse -- one theological and one linguistic. The key ideas of "word," "transformation," and "deep structure" need explaining.

In biblical theology, God is known as "The Word" (Genesis 1:1; John 1:1). The Greek word for "Word" is Logos. Logos refers to the order-creating and meaning-making force -- law or purpose or power or intelligence or principle as it is variously translated -- at work in the universe. Theologians linked the Old Testament meaning of the Word as God's self-disclosure with the philosophical meaning of Logos as controlling principle to refer particularly to Jesus as the Christ, the Logos and Wisdom of God (Harvey 1964, 146-148; Richardson and Bowden 1983, 338-339).

In linguistics, "Word" has a different meaning. Linguists who use a "transformational grammar" model of language identify two levels in the structure of language: (1) Surface Structure, which determines how the parts of a sentence go together in every sentence of each particular language, and (2) Deep Structure which gives a complete representation of the meaning of a sentence (Bandler and Grinder 1975).

In this linguistic view, all surface words -- which mean language itself -- are transformations of the deep structure of reality as reality is represented fully in itself. In deep structure there is no representation of reality, there is only reality. In that transformation from deep structure to surface structure, information is deleted, distorted, and generalized, with the result that "words" are actually "maps" or "models" of the territory of deep structure and never the territory itself (Korzybski 1933).

The linguistic view of reality as deep structure reflects the old mammalian brain in my opinion. There in the subcortical region we are encountering both an outer world and our own inner world. It is presentational reality prior to conceptualization. It is the realm Polanyi called "the tacit dimension" (Polanyi 1966), the base of "personal knowledge" (Polanyi [1958] 1964), the locus of spontaneous intuitive integration which works in tandem with "the deliberately active powers of the imagination" (Polanyi 1968).

Words, thereby, are mental representations -- images and schemata which re-present experience. That re-presentation of experience enables us to convey to one another the meaning of what is happening to us. From a linguistic perspective the deep Word appears in and through our surface words. From a theological perspective "the deep word" is an analogical way of talking about God as "The Word." That is how interpretations take on the certainty of absolute explanation. Our stories become interpretive statements of what we regard as Real.

When we explain the meaning of our lives we express what we believe to be the truth of life. These beliefs constitute the ways by which we orient ourselves to the world and the ways in which we organize the world. We know who we are by the stories we tell. We know how to act because of the ideas we share. In short, our words give voice to The Word that makes life meaningful.

I would like to present two ideas from philosopher Paul Ricouer (1978) and theologian David Tracy (1981, 202-229, 376-389, 398-404) that express convictions about the presence of God. One is called "the hermeneutics of proclamation;" the other "the phenomenology of manifestation." Proclamation deals with saving the world, while manifestation expresses savoring the world. These two theological ideas are generalizations made from the stories of our lives as people of faith.

.

Saving the World: Proclamation

The interpretive activity in which we all engage carries the technical label of "hermeneutics." We shape what we perceive according to the cognitive maps we make of the external world. In making those maps we combine bodily perception with imaginative construction for the sake of articulated meaning (Johnson 1987).

Thus, in the Judeo-Christian tradition, proclamation has involved interpreting what people have experienced primarily in terms of the pivotal events of Exodus and Easter. The focus is on the Word which emerges from the awesome presence of the Wholly Other (Ricouer 1978, 21). The Exodus story frees us from the drag of the past by confronting us with the possibilities in freedom. At the same time Easter frees us from the dread of the future by opening before us the actuality of destiny (Ashbrook 1971, 77-86; Ashbrook and Walaskay 1977, 106). In telling of these events we are interpreting who we are in our humanity (Golding 1981 and 1982, 46-47, 60).

Story-telling results in meaning-making, and meaning-making leads to formal theology. Experience becomes organized around basic speech acts: telling stories, giving instruction, and affirming doctrine. The way things appear on the surface is regarded with suspicion. What truly matters is the unseen, that which cannot be discerned by the eye alone, namely, transcendent truth as known in narrated reality (Goldberg 1981 and 1982, 194-240). Humanity lives in a condition of distortion and misperception. Life's true order has not yet been realized. God judges the fallen world -- society, humanity, nature, and even the cosmos itself -- in order to transform and redeem it.

The Christian tradition abounds with world-transforming expressions: prophetic witness, proclamation of the kerygma as Good News, the Protestant Principle, the Word-Event, the crucified Christ, the eschatological future, doctrine, dogma. We find no neat separation between Protestant and Catholic expressions in regard to the deceptiveness of appearances. Thomas Aquinas stated the issue in a way which Tillich identified as "argumentative rationality": "The human intellect cannot reach by natural virtue the divine substance, because, according to the way of the present life the cognition of our intellect starts with the senses" (quoted by Tillich 1959, 16, 18).

Each of these expressions point to political, ethical, rational, or historical elements. They share the common feature of a critical judgment on reality as ordinarily perceived. The world in which we live is viewed as limited and limiting. Any aesthetic appreciation is rejected in favor of conceptualized interpretations and ethical imperatives. In the recital of a history of liberation from bondage, this emphasis minimizes, and actually dismisses, the rhythmic patterns of the natural world.

Proclamation is word-oriented. People hear the truth and are to act on the basis of that truth. In the Old Testament we find the repeated formula: "Hear, O Israel . . ." In the New Testament Jesus declares: "You have heard it said . . .but I say unto you . . ." We are called upon to be obedient to what is urgently right. Explicit explanation has been abstracted from unarticulated experience. Whatever bodily imagination has contributed to the formulation of what matters has crystallized into precise language.

Whether in a dynamic of suspicion about the human situation or in a static certainty about the truth of the Gospel, proclamation means "Hear! and believe! Save the world from itself!"

Savoring the World: Manifestation

In contrast to proclamation, manifestation lifts up the very features of life which word-oriented beliefs tend to minimize. Here we find the rhythmic process of the natural order -- the sun and the stars, the sea and the soil, the rain and the rainbow, the snow and the blossoming. All elicit from us a sense of wonder in the presence of the overwhelming power of what is surely and truly "given." Such mysteries never pass over "completely into articulation" (Ricouer 1978, 21). We babble on about them without ever containing them.

In other words, we experience the world itself as the center of the really real. A rock, a mountain, a tree, a ritual, an archetype, an icon, a myth each conveys and affirms the power of Immanent Reality. We know the graciousness of God in what is immediately tangible. That may be in the experience of our body with its sensuality and sexual reality. That may be in our relationship with others through experiences of the communal, the traditional, and social reality. That may be in our immersion in the nonhuman world of the natural, the ecological, and the mystical that gives a certainty of cosmic reality. We have been created in the image and likeness of what truly is, already known and always being realized. The experience of God's love calls us to affirm nature and to affirm life, wholly good and wholly one.

As with proclamation, the Christian tradition abounds with expressions of this world-affirming creative power: sacramental presence, apologetic theology, Catholic Substance, the incarnation and resurrection, realized eschatology, "the feeling of absolute dependence" (Schleiermacher 1958). Despite his struggle with a fallen view of creation, Augustine voiced this experience of manifestation in what Tillich (1959, 16) called "an immediate rationality": "Where I found Truth, there found I my God, who is the Truth" (Augustine 1955, BK. X, XXIV, 222-223). Each of these expressions conveys a sense of the esthetic or mystical, a mystery which is already and always present and active. They all share the quality of finding the extraordinary in the midst of the ordinary. The concrete, tangible, physical world of appearance manifests -- shows forth and discloses -- the whole of what matters in the making of meaning.

Such religious expression is oriented to objects, appearances, the anchoring of imagination and meaning in bodily experience. The world vibrates with a sense of the numinous. Natural symbolic meaning blossoms. In the ecstatically intense language of Gerard Manley Hopkins' poem "God's Grandeur":

> The world is charged with the grandeur of God
> It will flame out, like shining from shook foil;
> It gathers to a greatness, like the ooze of oil
> Crushed. Why do men then now not reck his rod?
> Generations have trod, have trod, have trod;
> And all is seared with trade; bleared, smeared
> with toil;
> And wears man's smudge and shares man's smell: the
> soil
> Is bare now, nor can foot feel, being shod.
>
> And for all this, nature is never spent;
> There lives the dearest freshness deep down
> things;
> And though the last lights off the black West went
> Oh, morning, at the brown brink eastward, springs --
> Because the Holy Ghost over the bent
> World broods with warm breast and with ah! bright
> wings (Gardner [1953] 1958, 27).

(In order to experience the vivid power of the poem you might read it aloud three or four times with a different emphasis each time.)

Despite our human frailty and our human failure, "nature is never spent." "The world is charged with the grandeur of God . . .the Holy Ghost over the bent/World broods with warm breast" "[t]here lives the dearest freshness deep down things."

We can never say enough about such Reality. Yet we sing and celebrate, we dance and shout, we pray and praise. In the Old Testament that sacredness finds voice in the psalmist's litany of joy: "The heavens declare the glory of God, the vault of heaven proclaims God's handiwork" (Psalm 19:1 JB). Similarly, in the New Testament we are caught up in mystical wonder: "Ever since

God created the world God's everlasting power and deity -- however invisible -- have been there for the mind to see in the things God has made" (Romans 1:20 JB). We trust what is ultimately real. We experience the wholeness of God in the immediacy of every part of our world.

Whether in a dynamic espousal of the human situation or in a static confidence about the goodness of creation, manifestation means "O taste and see that the Lord is good (Psalm 34:8a)! Celebrate! Savor the world!"

Caring for the World: Prophetic Action

Through the centuries people have tended to emphasize one moment of the dialectic of religious experience in contrast to the other. For some, proclamation for the sake of transforming what is not right into what is urgently right has dominated. The story has been told in order to save the world. For others, manifestation and the affirmation of the really real has dominated. The story has been a celebrating of everything in the universe.

Most people, however, like Second Isaiah, have held saving and savoring together. They have combined stories of freedom with stories of fulfillment. Creating meant redeeming and redeeming meant creating. No affirmation without transformation, no tranformation without affirmation. Only our double mind, with the analyzing and explaining power of the left hemisphere, divides indivisible reality. God is the God of all -- everyone and everything, even those people and those things we do not like. Biblical scholar James A. Sanders identifies this understanding as "monotheizing," the disturbing insistence by the biblical authors that God as God creates and sustains all of creation (Sanders 1987b).

In recent years the prophetic care of the world has moved beyond an artificial dialectic or dichotomy between saving and savoring. What is real and right has merged into that which is trustworthy and true. Both the visible and the invisible, the physical and the purposeful, the bodily and the imaginative, the sensory and the symbolic draw upon and require each other. That concern with making real what is right has surfaced in what Tracy calls prophetic/action-oriented theology (Tracy 1981, 371, 390-398, 431, 434-437). I am not alone in calling it "caring for the world." It is exercising responsibility for the world in which we find ourselves (Genesis 1:26).

In the first half of the twentieth century a heightened sensitivity to the suffering caused by injustice emerged in The Social Gospel Movement. Out of his own deep evangelical piety, Walter Rauschenbusch (1909) voiced the social crisis of his time (1912), directed attention to the imperative of "Christianizing the Social Order" (1913), and articulated a full "Theology for the Social Gospel" (1919). The collapse of western optimism with World War I, and what Friedrick Nietzsche called "The Death of God," namely, the breakdown of the assumptions upon which our modern world was based, exposed the shallowness of a rationalistic prophetic imperative. Proclamation and manifestation, the universal and the particular appeared to be opposed to each other as only an interpretive left brain would assume.

However, the potential conflict between traditional proclamation and traditional manifestation is receding. In its place we are discovering what Tracy identifies as "a fidelity to the concrete" situations of suffering and systemic bondage (Tracy 1981, 392; see Chopp 1986). Liberation and political theologies avoid the artificial distinction between proclamation and manifestation, between imperative and indicative, between transforming what is unjust and affirming what is trustworthy, between saving and savoring. Such praxis is prophetic, action-oriented and pragmatic. How do we live the story of meaning-making so that it becomes everybody's story?

I suggest that such caring about the world arises more from a prophetic mysticism than from prophetic action alone. By prophetic mysticism I mean that deep structure of meaning-making that protests oppressive principalities and powers

(Ephesians 6:12) in the power of that which liberates humanness. In terms of evolutionary theory, selective pressure is on the side of optimal adaptational responses for the species as a whole and never for only part of the species (Burhoe 1981).

Political theologies are theologies of protest in specific historical situations. Belief incorporates the imperative of transforming the world. Liberation theologies are theologies of promise in specific historical moments. Belief draws upon the indicative of affirming the world. Together, saving and savoring are strategies of caring for that which is just in society and true in community. Together, saving and savoring are ways of caring for the world by exposing the contradictions of the dominant culture. Together, saving and savoring are approaches of caring for the world that shift faith and practice from concern with personal alienation to concentration on political oppression -- "economic dependency, sexism, racism, classism, elitism" (Tracy 1981, 394). Prophetic belief means pragmatic action -- caring for the world in ways that make a difference. Caring for the world seeks to transform "what is given" in terms of "what God is about." What we do arises from where we are.

Summary

I have sketched ways in which people have discerned the meaning of what matters in life. Some organize their experience in terms of saving the world. That is known as God's redeeming and tranforming activity or what calls for saving the world. Others give themselves to the experience of God's creating and affirming activity or what invites a savoring of the world. Still others, out of a radical immersion in the immediacy of their own cultural crippling, give expression to God's liberating activity or what can be called caring for the world. In contrast to the dialectic between proclamation and manifestation, caring for the world -- prophetic action -- embodies, envisions, and engages God's liberating activity.

Patterns of belief -- whether distinguishable or combined with one another -- express our perceptions of that Reality at work in the human reality that we are and in the physical reality of which we are a part. Similarly, ways in which our brain works -- whether a left brain rationality or a right brain relationality -- express our involvement in that Reality at work in the physical reality that we are and in the purposive reality of which we are the exemplar -- the old mammalian and reptilian cortices.

We can speak of the brain in terms of "mind," by which I refer to the human meaning of the brain, namely, all the social, cultural, artistic, religious, political activity which characterizes the presence of humanity.

We can speak of mind in terms of "brain," by which I refer to the materiality of the mind, namely, the biochemical processes without which we humans do not function.

Finally, we can speak of God as that power which creates a meaningful world and makes us a reality in that world. Reality, quite simply, is another name for God -- "I am that I am," "I cause to be what comes into being," "I will be what I will be," YHWH (Exodus 3:14). Unlike "a thing" which has reached its final form, God is Nameless Name -- the "name of four letters" without vowels -- Living Reality (Anderson 1962b; Abba 1962; Ashbrook 1971, 25-27; Fromm 1966, 31). The deep Word of all surface words is The Word which is Reality, and that Reality is Word -- the Logos of meaning making.

In the language of the biblical witness, the human species is made "in the image and likeness of God" (Genesis 1:26-28). Without that image and likeness nothing exists. With that image and likeness everything exists. We are meaning-making creatures precisely because we embody that Reality which makes meaning meaningful. This is the story -- the belief -- of our lives! We believe we are "at home!"

CHAPTER EIGHT

PATTERNS OF BELIEF

Bless the Lord, O my soul;
and all that is within me,
bless [God's] holy name!
(Psalm 103:1 RSV)

As far back in history as we can go, people have disagreed about what makes us human (Kolb and Whishaw [1980] 1985, 304). Human beings were more than the sum of their parts, yet various parts conveyed the sense of their humanness. Was the core some particular part of us -- body, bowels, heart, head -- or some particular quality in us -- breath, feeling, thought, will, soul? Among the Greeks, some located the part in the heart, while others thought of the head. The Hebrews present a more complex picture of bodily parts and metaphorical images of what it means to be human (Wolff 1974, 7-79). Regardless of what or where, all that is within us adds up to our being more than simply ourselves.

But what is the connection between the wonder of ourselves and the wonder of our world? How are the widest reaches of belief linked with the narrower processes that subserve the patterns which convey the deep convictions about the nature of our reality?

Brain versus Heart

Among the Greeks, Empedocles (ca. 490-430 B.C.E.) and Aristotle (384-322 B.C.E.) developed what could be called the cardiac hypothesis -- deciding "that because the heart was warm and active it was the source of mental processes." Alcaeon of Croton (ca. 500 B.C.E.) and Plato (420-347 B.C.E.), in contrast, subscribed to what is now known as the brain hypothesis -- placing the rational part of a tripartite soul "in the brain because that was the part of the body closest to the heavens." As physicians, Hippocrates (430-379 B.C.E.) and Galen (129-199 C.E.) argued for the brain hypothesis.

Despite the scientific inaccuracy of the cardiac hypothesis as the locus of the human, "the heart" metaphor persists. The biblical writers believed the heart represented "the innermost spring of individual life, the ultimate source of all its physical, intellectual, emotional, and volitional energies, and consequently the part of [a human being] through which [one] normally achieved contact with the divine" (Denton 1962, 549-550). As the prophet Jeremiah expressed the assumption: "Behold, the days are coming, says the Lord, when I will make a new covenant with the house of Israel and the house of Judah . . . I will put my law within them, and I will write it upon their hearts" (Jeremiah 31:31-34 RSV). The heart of God was the organ which most conveyed the will of God -- God's inclination toward humanity and God's capacity for mercy (Wolff 1974, 55-58):

> My people . . . how could I give you up? . . .
> My heart recoils from it,
> my whole being trembles at the thought.
> I will not give rein to my fierce anger, . . .
> For I am God and not [humanity] . . .
> I . . . have no wish to destroy.
> (Hosea 11:7-9 JB)

Although "heart" conveys compassion, "head" provides clues as how to carry out that divine mercy. "Brain" is a metaphor for God in as much as it is not God -- nor is any other part of creation, as Augustine expressed so powerfully. But once we recognize every expression of God is a metaphor the next step becomes transforming the metaphor into an analogy -- a similarity between the part and the whole, a continuity between the way we are put together and the way God puts together the universe.

The metaphor of the brain provides a more fruitful way to deepen our understanding of ourselves and the universe than the heart per se. In its actual functioning the heart is an organ, a replaceable part as we now know is common in heart transplants. But the brain is not a replaceable part, even though parts of it are now repairable as in fetal transplant for specific deficiency like Parkinson's disease. As a prime metaphor of meaning, the brain provides specific understanding of how the whole brain can function for the sake of the whole human family.[1]

Jesus summons us to love God, our neighbor, and ourselves "with all" our heart, soul, mind, and strength (Mark 12:29-31). These were the two great commandments, and in stating them in this form he added to the original commandment (Deuteronmy 6:4) the word "mind." Together the images and ideas of heart, soul, mind, and strength create a configuration of human wholeness in its relationship to divine intention.

Consider each of those words in turn (Arndt and Gingrich [1958, 1957] 1979; Kittel 1964):

> love, which in Greek is agape, involves will and action, an intentional and intelligent cherishing of the wellbeing of others apart from one's own, a neighbor love which includes love of enemies in an unconditional way;

> heart, which in Greek is kardia, refers to our inner nature and character, the source and center of all the feelings and emotions, desires and passions, the organ of enlightenment, the dwelling place of heavenly disposition, the seat of the will which determines moral conduct;

> soul, which in Greek is psyche, indicates living being, the physical life which is the center of the inner life in its many and varied aspects that transcend the earthly;

> mind, or the Greek word dianoia, means intentional purpose, thought, plan, disposition, understanding; and

strength, the translation for the Greek <u>ischuous</u>, means physical, mental, or spiritual ability and power to concentrate on the love of God.

In addition, in *The Book of Romans* St. Paul suggests how that imperative might be followed, namely: ". . . let your mind be renewed and your whole nature thus transformed . . ." (Romans 12:2 NEB). Here the word mind, or in Greek <u>nous</u>, indicates the whole person. Mind refers to the capacity of thinking in contrast to physical existence and thereby refers to the higher mental part of the natural, person which, as the sum total of the whole mental and moral condition of every person, initiates thoughts and plans. And the word transformed -- <u>metamorphosis</u> -- refers to a revolution in one's thinking which brings with it a new moral sensitivity in which what is invisible to the physical eye becomes outwardly visible in one's total functioning.

Most of all, however, in advancing the metaphor of brain -- or mind since I am using these terms synonymously -- the Greek word <u>kardia</u> in the New Testament refers to the faculty of thought, of the thoughts themselves, of understanding, of the organ of natural and spiritual enlightenment. In this area, **kardia** may often be, and often is, translated as "mind" instead of "heart."[2] The brain thereby suggests mechanisms with which we can understand the heart of humanity.

With this new understanding of the processes which underlie belief we can mobilize energy in more constructive ways. With this new understanding we can activate imagination in more creative ways. With this new understanding we can be more like the way we have been created to be. Knowledge of the brain can transform our mind's beliefs into that which is more than simply "appealing figures of speech" (Ehrenwald 1986, 274).

We can know the mechanisms of our making of meaning and we can use that knowledge for the whole human family, the whole family of God, the whole firmament which is our home. As we know the brain, so we know the wonder of ourselves and the wonder of the world of which we are a part (Psalm 139:14).

To that goal of more practical faith and more faithful practice I draw together the distinguishable threads of brain, mind, and belief into a more systematic form. Brain science alone does not -- and cannot -- capture the significance of human life. No physiological process adequately accounts for human purposing. Cognitive science alone does not -- and cannot -- evaluate the values with which we engage life. No mental representation adequately accounts for human presence. Nor do belief patterns alone create the conditions which make for life. No cosmic consciousness adequately accounts for human behavior. But together, brain activity and belief patterns, as mediated in cognitive processes, provide a convergence of the crucial features with which we can engage faith and action.

To love "with all" our mind, therefore, requires that we utilize all our brain. We are to "put on the new nature, created after the likeness of God" (Ephesians 4:24). We now know that the brain consists of different depths of complexity, different patterns of processing information, different combinations of tension-and-relaxation, with each performing different functions in different ways as part of the whole-making process. We now know that all parts are necessary for thinking, feeling, and acting. Without the contribution of every part, the whole disintegrates into a broken brain, a troubled mind, or an oppressive belief (Ashbrook 1987).

Just as we know there is a biochemical individuality (Williams 1956) as unique as our fingerprints, so we know there is an individuality in the brain that is equally unique. Every brain is an individual brain; there is no such entity as a universal brain. To put the issue sharply: there are only brains -- plural, not singular. Thus, despite our pursuit of regularities of human life, we always find ourselves in the presence of a holy of holies in which every predicted pattern can be dissolved in the crucible of an immediate context.

In the fullness of life we always experience the flowing of life -- grace in theological terms, optimal adaptation in evolutionary terms. In the stunted caricature of life we always stumble into the constriction of life -- sin in theological terms, adaptational dysfunction in evolutionary terms. The task becomes that of encouraging the flow and minimizing the constriction. To that end I advance a mapping of believing brains, an overview of the territory of human meaning-making.

Maps have value when we need direction. They get in the way when we substitute the map for the territory. The following map of the believing brain is intended to serve two purposes: (1) to encourage our cosmos-making propensity, and (2) to reduce our cosmos-destroying capacity.

I provide three kinds of map -- a visual summary in Figure 8; a verbal summary in Table 6; a synthesizing diagram in Figure 9. I describe the analysis in the text itself. These maps assume three dimensions:

the conspicuous anatomical division and functional specialization *between* the hemispheres, that is, the left (dominant) mind with its logical detailed representation of proclamation, or what matters eternally, and the right (nondominant) mind with its symbolic imagination of manifestation, or what matters tangibly;

the less conspicuous functional divisions *within* each hemisphere, that is, receptive input from the posterior (back) regions -- contextual sensitivity by the right brain and content abstraction by the left brain -- and active output from the anterior (front) regions -- imaginative construction by the right brain and systematic focus by the left brain;

and finally, *below the level of consciousness*, the master coordinating region of the limbic system -- the emotional mind -- with its sensitive reciprocity with both the felt-meaning of the immediate environment and long term evolutionary developments.

When put together, these three dimensions of brain activity form a map of patterns of belief. At the level of consciousness -- the neocortex -- I identify two major families of resemblance (proclamation and manifestation), each with two variations.[3] Below consciousness -- in the old mammalian brain -- I locate what is called prophetic action. I describe each in detail to show how the brain can be used in understanding not only how we perceive ourselves but also how we perceive our life with God (See Figure 8).

In various times and among various people we find a preference for one of these configurations of belief over other configurations. In most mature believers, however, the preference includes what is emphasized in the other aspects of belief. Only in disturbed belief do we find a fixation of one kind of processing to the exclusion of the other processes.

Left Brain Belief: Saving the World

A preference for belief in a left brain mode of consciousness emphasizes "saving" the world. People believe that God entrusts them with responsibility for the created order. So, they name every "thing" that is, and they analyze the validity of all they take to be reality. To proclaim redemption means to declare what life is about for the sake of saving it.

Those who are predisposed to the redemptive pattern regard life as a pilgrimage. In order to live toward a fulfillment yet-to-be realized (Psalm 68, Ephesians 4:18), like Abraham and Sarah, they go out from an enmeshed Ur of the Chaldeans (Hebrews 11) or are delivered from an oppressive bondage (Exodus). Like Abraham and Sarah, they live in the Promised Land as strangers and foreigners -- outsiders -- living in tents -- on the road -- looking forward to a reality beyond the realities around them (Hebrews 11:8-16).

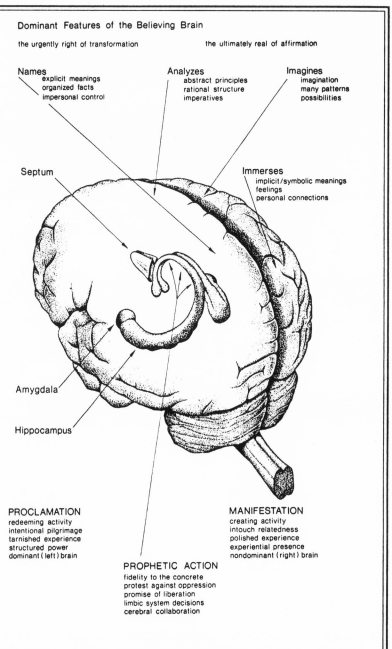

Dominant Features of the Believing Brain

the urgently right of transformation   the ultimately real of affirmation

Names
    explicit meanings
    organized facts
    impersonal control

Analyzes
    abstract principles
    rational structure
    imperatives

Imagines
    imagination
    many patterns
    possiblilities

Septum

Immerses
    implicit/symbolic meanings
    feelings
    personal connections

Amygdala

Hippocampus

PROCLAMATION
redeeming activity
intentional pilgrimage
tarnished experience
structured power
dominant (left) brain

MANIFESTATION
creating activity
intouch relatedness
polished experience
experiential presence
nondominant (right) brain

PROPHETIC ACTION
fidelity to the concrete
protest against oppression
promise of liberation
limbic system decisions
cerebral collaboration

FIGURE 8. Limbic System and Mechanisms of Belief.

The logic of proclamation leads them to reject immediate values. Whether those values are values of nature (Isaiah 44:9-20), or values of family (Matthew 10:34-36), or values of the institutions of government (Deuteronomy 5:2-3) and religion (Jeremiah 7:1-11; Hebrews 9:1-14; Revelation 21:22), the logic of proclamation leads them to reject such immediate values as limiting. The hermeneutic of suspicion always raises question about the sustaining value of every finite vessel. There is value in earthen vessels, but every vessel is *"earthen"* -- limited and limiting when it becomes an end in itself (2 Corinthians 4:7).

Left brain orientation always reflects a distance from the immediate situation. It observes what is happening from above and outside -- an Olympian perspective to use a metaphor from Greek mythology. That very distance cuts one off from the full resources within the context. By virtue of that separation, we neutralize experiencel at best and tarnished it at worst. Triggered at the limbic level by the emergency reactions of the sympathetic system's perception of threat to the survival of the self, the emotional arousal minimizes positive features, stabilizes neutral features, and exaggerates negative features. In its most adaptive form the excitement empowers us to contact and use the things of this world for the sake of the things that matter most.

All relationships must be righted in obedience to what is still to come (Jenni 1962).

Naming

In its receptive functioning, a left mind belief "names" what is there. We find that pattern in Genesis 2:19-20 (JB) where Yahweh God brings all the wild beasts and birds before Adam "to see what he would call them; each one was to bear the name the man would give it." The scenerio places humanity at the center of the world (Genesis 2:4b-3:24; Ashbrook 1973, 146).

We live in an anthropocentric universe. Even though we are not the last word about life, our presence constitutes the central fact of our life. We interpret reality exclusively in terms of human values and human experience. We find that fact in the metaphorical and imaginative foundation of language (Lakoff and Johnson 1980). Every experience occurs within a context of cultural presuppositions. We transform emergent metaphors, such as "happy means to be up," into concepts related to other terms, such as health, life, goodness, and movement (Lakoff and Johnson 1980, 58).

Labels make for easier reference even as they give objects reality. The name tag takes on an independent existence. Images turn into ideas. We replace impressions with descriptions. We make things orderly; we organize according to maps or models in our head; we arrange things conceptually. That means everything is capable of having referential existence. We indicate something as being a focus of attention. In short, we live in a "named" reality.

Thus, objects are given explicit meaning. That seeming objectivity contributes to our taking our abstract map for the actual territory. What we can define we regard as definitive. We objectify the configuration of bodily experience and imagination (Johnson 1987; Lakoff 1987). We transform these configurations -- prototypes in technical language -- into substantial and permanent entities. Our ability to name marks the unique advance in evolution from strictly mammalian complexity to human complexity. "In the Beginning Was the 'Name,'" as psychologist H.S. Terrace phrases it (Terrace 1985).

Other mammals interact with their environment through smell and sight. They neither name objects nor refer to them abstractly. In teaching apes to use American Sign Language as the mode of communicating with us, researchers have found that the symbolic capacity of apes is primarily imitative and nonspontaneous (Terrace 1985). There is no evidence that apes, nor any other mammal, intend to convey information for any other than immediate instrumental purposes. They do not transmit information for its own sake. Apes lack "an understanding of the fact that one can refer to an object by its name" (Terrace 1985, 1021) alone.

In contrast, by "naming" objects we shift our sensory preference to the vocal and verbal, the abstract and intentional. We can delight in contemplating an object for its own sake. We can savor sharing that perception of an object -- like a sunset or a symphony or a special scotch -- with another person. The capacity to develop a focus, to intend a mutual attention to some particular aspects of the world, has been given the technical terms of "proto-imperative" and "proto-declarative" (Bates 1976, cited by Terrace 1985, 1019). We signal to one another by words, by gestures, and by glances that there is "something to look at." And there is "something to look at" precisely because we designate that in the midst of "everything" there is "some 'thing'."

One of the most powerful effects of the phenomenon of "naming" is the activation of a shared world. In the metaphor of the Garden myth, Yahweh asks Adam to refer to objects by name. Here is the prototype of the delight of a parent and a child seeing "a spoon" or "a doggie" or "a bottle" eye-to-eye, together, creating a known world, that is, "naming" reality. What matters in the moment is not what we "do" with the named thing, but rather that we "notice" the thing named (Terrace 1985, 1026). Sheer intrinsic value, value for its own sake, valued for our knowing together!

That specific, however, can lose the context out of which "naming" arises and in which it prospers. The left half can ignore the right half. Words replace Word; things replace "thous," to coin a phrase from Martin Buber. The map obliterates the territory. Instead of loving people and using things, as Reuel Howe put it, we find ourselves "using people and loving things" (Howe 1953). Obedience to the shared relationship turns into compulsion to keep every "thing" in its place, as it "is" according to our "naming" it. Controlling the environment takes over from our caring for the world.

Even though we can reduce the "naming" aspect of belief to literalism, the fact that we can share in creating a world -- a cosmos, a named reality -- both reflects and contributes to our being "made in the image and likeness of God" (Genesis 1:26). That truth is neither far from us nor hard to know. As Moses told the children of Israel in the desert:

> It is not in heaven, that you should say, "Who will go up for us to heaven, and bring it to us, that we may hear it and do it?" Neither is it beyond the sea, that you should say, "Who will go over the sea for us, and bring it to us, that we may hear it and do it?" But the word is very near you; it is in your mouth and in your heart, so that you can do it (Deuteronomy 30:11-14 RSV).

Analyzing

We never simply "name" reality; we go on to analyze reality. What is the truth of the situation? Or as 1 John admonishes us: "Do not believe every spirit, but test the spirits to see whether they are of God" (1 John 4:1 RSV). Our believing brains not only receive and perceive "what is," we are also wired to conceive and construct "what ought to be."

In its active functioning, a left mind "analyzes" what ought to be. That "ought to be" means conforming to the will of God, the Lord of history, those conditions necessary for optimal evolutionary adaptation, in short, to what is right for us and every living creature in our relatedness to each other. While such "ought to be" represents an ideal toward which we strive, it actually constitutes what is given in our very existence. Thus the orientation can be understood as analytical and systematic. It abstracts underlying principles or features and then develops them systematically into a rational structure of explanation and accountability.

Remember the response of the split brain patient Paul who casually answered the inquiry about his selection of the shovel along with the chicken head -- "we need the shovel to clean out the chicken shed." We may not always have our information straight, but we very well can make a case for the way we believe things to be. Among the many possible maps of the territory of belief, the left mind preference takes on compelling conviction. The picture is complete. It alone is right. In an analytical distinction between "good and bad," "right and wrong," "this and that," one part is taken to be more important than the other parts. As Nasrudin argued, the moon becomes more important than the sun. There is only one right way to fold our hands.

At its best, the analyzing aspect of the brain identifies and lives by that which matters most for genuinely human life. The biblical expression of this comes with the spelling out of the convenant between Yahweh God and the Children of Israel at Mount Sinai (Exodus 19ff; Leviticus) -- what is known as the Mosaic tradition (Mendenhall 1955). Regulations range from stealing and cursing to offering sacrifices and separating the clean from the unclean. These requirements were derived from the experience of people being accountable to God for the exercise of responsibility for their life in community.

Thus the Lord Yahweh shows Amos a vision of a man standing by a wall with a plumb-line in his hand: "Look, I am going to measure my people Israel by plumb-line; no longer will I overlook their offenses" (Amos 7:7-9 JB). We are to assess life as life is meant to be lived under God (Hosea 4:1-3). Because of the capacity of the left mind, in its active mode, faith and practice are freed from being enmeshed in any and every social structure. We are cultural creatures who are called to transform culture in light of the reality of God.

We are to approach life in an intentional way, analyzing facts in order to heighten that which matters most. Coherence emerges out of chaos. Direction appears as we stand on our feet and survey our world. We are meant to make the many meanings of our lives meaningful for the whole human family. Left minded belief redeems and reforms "what is" in accordance with what is supposed to be. I suggest that is the underlying process which results in the New Testament insisting:

Enter by the narrow gate, since the road that leads to
perdition is wide and spacious and many take it; but it is
a narrow gate and a hard road that leads to life, and only
a few find it (Matthew 7:13-14 JB).

For a vigilant, step-by-step strategy, it is abundantly clear that life
be urgently right. Faith is tested as people exert effort to control
chaos (Pierce 1986). The process makes us intend that reality for
which we are made.

Those who prefer a left brain belief emphasize saving the world.
They grab on to an orderly and idealized meaning of life. They insist that life is not for naught. Life makes sense, and we are to act
according to that sensibility. It is left brain activity which tries to
transform the world in terms of what we perceive to be the light of
God. In nonreligious language we can speak of that as conforming
to the laws of life, the ecosystem in which we find ourselves.

Right Brain Belief: Savoring the World

Consider now the pattern of a right brain preference. In this mode
of consciousness what matters is savoring the world. People
believe that God has created everything "good" and therefore
nothing in creation is to be depreciated. Thus, they are immersed
in the settings in which they find themselves, and they envision the
best of all possible worlds. To manifest creation means to savor
the life we know.

Those predisposed to the creation pattern engage life relationally.
Genesis 5:1 (JB) illustrates the orientation: "This is the roll of
Adam's [and Eve's] descendents . . ." Geneologies identify the supposed origins and recognized affinities among groups and individuals (Bowman 1962; Throckmorton 1962; Patton and Childs
1987). We come into this world, continue in this world, and die
only in relationship to a context that we neither originate nor control. We have only been entrusted with its care, not its mastery.
There is but one reality, one God, one context "from whom [or
which] all things come and for whom [or which] we exist," in the

same way as there is for Christians "one Lord, Jesus Christ, through whom all things come and through whom we exist" (1 Corinthians 8:5 JB).

The logic of manifestation includes everything and affirms everything. Whether these realities are the natural world (Psalm 103; Job 38ff), or realities of the family (Genesis 1:28; Deuteronomy 5:5; Ecclesiasticus 7:27-29), or realities of the institutions of government (2 Samuel 5:1-3; Mark 12:17; John 19:11; Romans 13:1-7) and religion (1 Corinthians 12:27), the logic of manifestation leads them to affirm every reality as valuable and necessary in and of itself. The hermeneutic of espousal locates us within the world, lifting up its intrinsic worth -- even the hairs on our head (Matthew 10:30) and the flowers and grass of the field (Matthew 6:25-33). There is value in earthen vessels, to return to the metaphor of left brain proclamation, and every vessel is *"treasure"* - - limitless and liberating when it is known in its relational reality, the context of care and connection.

A right brain orientation resonates with the immediate situation. It participates in what is happening from within -- a personal and personalizing presence. That very intimacy sensitizes us to the full resources within the context. By virtue of that resonance, experience becomes optimal adaptation at best and polished illusion at worst. Triggered at the limbic level by the relaxing responses of the parasympathetic system's perception of possibility in the continuity of life, emotional affinity with the context minimizes negative features, stabilizes pleasurable features, and exaggerates positive features. In its most adaptive form here is the energy which inspires us to synergistic openness to life and cooperation with reality in all its manifestations.

The whole world -- personal and nonpersonal -- vibrates with that which is ultimately real.

Immersing

In its receptive functioning, a right mind belief is "immersed" in a contextual universe in which it locates itself. We find that pattern in Genesis 1 where creation is a meaningful process because it takes place within a context of meaning. We can trust life's meaning because everything unfolds within the purposes of a reality with integrity (Sanders 1987b). Within that order the scenerio places humanity at the pinnacle of the creation pyramid (von Rad 1961, 48-49; Ashbrook 1973, 145).

To those of us who believe, we live in a theocentric universe. Even though we categorize life with the analytical tools of observing consciousness, things exist within a context. To create means to divide, and we can divide because we live in an integrated and integrating universe. Divisions exist: the right brain/the left brain; day/night; sun/moon, yet all come together -- all are joined together -- in their contexts because of the order out of which they emerge. The sun is not more important than the moon nor the moon more important than the sun. Rather, sun-and-moon together -- very good in all the reality of what is ultimately real. We order life, perhaps, in the way God "ordered" life.

The primary separation is the distinction between light and darkness, seeing from not seeing, consciousness from nonconsciousness (Ashbrook 1973, 145-146). The first experience of creation is not heaven and earth, but "light" -- "Let there be light" (Genesis 1:3). The initial awareness of Presence is illumination. Awareness of earth and sky, water and land, fish and birds, sun and moon, plants and animals follow. But in the experience of dawning -- discovering ourselves immersed in a context -- we know that we are made for the making of meaning.

Whether things fall into an order because we "see" their relatedness or because we "name" the order of related things is an unanswerable dilemma. What we do know is that we are co-creators in ordering reality in ways that are true and trustworthy. Our genes "give" us information about the environment of which we are a part. Our culture "creates" information about the world in which we live. Together, genes and culture combine in our imaging the ultimate values of our human universe.

That context is reflected in the response of the shepherds to the angelic host announcing the birth of a Saviour (Luke 2:8-20). In that unexpected event they make the strange phenomenon understandable by going to Bethlehem, the place associated with their Davidic tradition (Mendenhall 1955). Only then could they return to their own setting. Understanding required them to be "at home." Only then did they know what was going on.

Words, for instance, "convey information" as well as express and reinforce "the social structure" of which they are a part (Douglas [1970, 1973] 1982, 23). Every object bears symbolic meaning, which is dependent upon a person's knowing the particular context in which it exists. We live in a context of relationships which is cultural in its widest dimension and personal in its narrowest dimension.

Involvement requires some sense -- literally and not simply figuratively -- of trusting the world in which we find ourselves. A smile from one person to another "betokens" trust. So people came to believe that a rainbow in the sky is a sign of trust from God (Genesis 9:8-17).

That sense of relatedness, however, can lose a critical awareness of the order out of which "immersed" arises and from which it prospers. The right half can ignore the left half. Feelings then drown facts; the personal overpersonalizes everything. Trusting the differentiating process hardens into an uncritical assumption that "the way things appear" is "the way things are." Every contrast then constitutes a dualistic finality. Roles are "the" roles; rules are "the" rules; positions are "the" positions. The reality is less rational and more parochial, less conceptual and more cultural. Everything is concretized in a schizophrenic fantasy which takes immediate appearance for absolute reality.

Even though we can reduce the "immersed" aspect of belief to a parochial myopia, the fact we are aware of being part of a world -- a context of relatedness, an immersed reality -- both reflects and contributes to our being "made in the image and likeness of God" (Genesis 1:26). That truth is neither far from us nor hard to realize. As 1 John told the early Christians:

> It was there from the beginning; we have heard it; we have seen it with our own eyes; we looked upon it, and felt it with our own hands; and it is of this we tell. Our theme is the word of life. This life was made visible; we have seen it and bear our testimony; we here declare to you the eternal life which dwelt with the [Creator] and was made visible to us. What we have seen and heard we declare to you, so that you and we together may share in a common life, that life which we share with the [Creator] and [the Creator's] Son Jesus Christ. And we write this in order that the joy of us all may be complete (1 John 1:1-4 NEB).

Such conviction reflects the receptive processing of right brain activity. Our brain is wired to an orderly world because we are immersed in an ordering evolutionary environment.

Imagining

Unlike other mammals, we never simply are "immersed" in an environment. Because of the neocortex and the elaboration of the two hemispheres in their specialized contributions to cognitive activity, we always construct reality in a way which combines visceral perception with imaginative pattern making. At its core, pattern making consists of imaginative creations, finding and focusing in ever familiar and ever fanciful ways. Even the most abstract idea rests upon the metaphorical foundation of imagination (Lakoff and Johnson 1980; McFague 1982; 1987).

We think with our bodies and our bodies always exist within a milieu which is both visceral and perceptual (Johnson 1987).

"[N]onpropositional and figurative structures of embodied imagination" are central (Johnson 1987, xxxv) to our being and our knowing. Our brain not only experiences "what is," we are also wired to create "what might be." Theologian Sallie McFague refers to this representational process when she writes of "symbolic sensibility," "symbolic mentality," the necessity for "a metaphorical theology" (McFague 1982, 4-7).

In its initiating functioning a right mind "imagines" possibilities. That makes the orientation creative. Anything is imaginable, and thereby believable. Furthermore, everything holds together because everything flows from a coherent mind-set. The many patterns constitute variations on a symphonic theme of inspired hope. Imaginative belief affirms life in the present and life in the future (1 John 3:2).

Think of experiences that evoke some of our strongest emotions: beauty is one; joy another; hope still another. Whether these emotions provoke the positiveness of the right brain or the right brain embodies these emotions is an unanswerable dichotomy. What we do know is that the right brain, as an extension of the limbic system, "reads" the world in terms of its emotional meaning. Pleasure, cooperation, responsive caring come when the parasympathetic nervous system gives priority to relaxed excitement in contrast to tense uncertainty. The experience of pleasure in the presence of something beautiful -- as expressed on a human face in the form of a smile -- comes from the warm transaction between stimulus from the outside world and receptivity on the part of the person's inner reality.

In savoring what is manifested in the world we find an openness to life. We live in a future fulfillment which "has come" (1 Corinthians 10:11); we have "tasted the goodness of the word of God and the powers of the age to come" (Hebrews 6:5). In technical terms, theology calls this fulfillment "realized eschatology," the reality in which God is already present and at work (Richardson and Bowden 1983, 184-185). Specifically, with the belief -- the perception -

- that God is at work in every situation people are more relaxed than tense, more attentive to receive information from the world around them as well as from the world inside them. They are capable of imagining what makes for life instead of being haunted by what hinders life.

An imaginative mode of belief keeps life fresh. Everything is filled with promise and all-embracing (Moltmann 1967). We can see and sense the "might be" of what is made to be meaningful. We live for an ever expanding awareness of God as we attempt to discover who we are in the universe in which we live.

To the eye of faith life is never a dead end. Rather, life is lived in a reality of metanoia -- the Greek word for change -- a turn-about -- a reframing. As theologian H. Richard Niebuhr once defined the Good News: we can reinterpret every interpretation. In the imagery of the Psalmist, stones which builders reject turn out to be cornerstones (Psalm 118:22-23). What was useless to ordinary consciousness is transformed by the imaginative alchemy of faith into something usable. Dead ends mark new beginnings.

Much of the biblical material becomes plausible in light of the brain processes which seem to underlie patterns of belief. So a Joseph could inform his brothers who had schemed against him, thrown him into an abandoned well to get rid of him, and then found him to be the second most powerful person in Egypt: "Fear not . . . you meant evil against me; but God meant it for good . . ." (Genesis 50:19-20). Or, in the powerful words of St. Paul:

> It is plain to anyone with eyes to see that at the present time all created life groans in a sort of universal travail. And it is plain, too, that we who have a foretaste of the Spirit are in a state of painful tension . . . in our moments of impatience let us remember that hope always means waiting for something that we do not yet possess .
> . .

The Spirit of God not only maintains this hope within us, but helps us in our present limitations . . . we know that to those who love God, who are called according to [God's] plan, everything that happens fits into a pattern for good (Romans 8:22-28 Phillips).

Notice the realistic references in this material: "you meant evil against me" and "life groans . . . a state of painful tension . . . moments of impatience." These reflect the contribution of the left hemisphere with its observing vigilance. Yet the realism is absorbed into a right hemisphere pattern of meaning making: "but God meant it for good" and "a foretaste of the Spirit." Help in "present limitations" comes from the right brain imagining inconceivable -- inconceivable because the left brain only processes a step-at-a-time -- possibilities for good.

When St. Paul writes that for those "who are called according to [God's] plan, everything that happens fits into a pattern for good" (Romans 8:28 Phillips), he is drawing upon the capacity of the limbic system for optimal evolutionary adaptation in the face of any kind of obstacle. Left brain realism is incorporated into right brain responsiveness. We live in a universe which makes creative meaning a realistic possibility.

Such hope does not mean everything which happens "is good." Nor does it mean anything which comes is the intentional act of God. Rather, it means that -- "made in the image of God" as we are -- we can create inconceivable possibilities in even the most hopeless situation, even in a criminal's cross in a city garbage dump (Luke 23:33).

Not everything is caused directly by God yet God participates in all that is and is to be. Because we live in a universe in which we are co-makers of meaning, nothing is ever finally fixed and finished. We have the capacity to re-present every conception of "the way things are."

The fourteenth century mystic Meister Eckhart (1260-1327) put the limitless possibilities of human life this way: "God never tied [our] salvation to any pattern. Whatever possibilities inhere in any pattern of life inhere in all, because God has given it so and denied it to none" (Blakney [1941] 1957, 288).

What we are learning about the brain gives credence to Eckhart's conviction about possibilities. The brain is wired to patterning possibilities. Unformed feelings and unvoiced images are processed through the right hemisphere in a way which makes them conscious. Once they are conscious the left hemisphere is in a position to transform them into words. Then we are able to say what we know subsymbolically in the old cortex -- that we are made for evolutionary continuity -- and to mean what we say symbolically in the new cortex -- that our origin is our destiny. The higher level of complexity in culture still must conform to the requirements given in the system of the cosmos.

Some such mechanisms as these must underlie the Christian experience of Jesus as the Christ of God. The belief reflects a predominantly right brain vision of what matters most in human life. This new covenant -- we might almost say metaphorically a second rainbow in the sky following the initial rainbow after the flood (Genesis 9:8-17) -- represented a mental re-presentation of the possibility of making "a new heaven and a new earth" (Revelation 21:1) here and now. A right brain context of what is meaningful re-patterns a left brain content of what makes up that meaning.

This imagination was so exciting in its initial breakthrough -- with its vision of community, trust, and care of human beings as precious in the sight of God, a pleasurable and relaxing response reflecting the activity of the parasympathetic nervous system -- that if everyone were converted on the spot all the world would change; the millenium would occur; a new heaven and a new earth would appear.

The excitement of that vision of a new life did indeed gird those early Christians who suffered persecution because of their faith. That their faith seemed to sustain them even in the Roman Colosseum can only testify to the power of their mental representation of what mattered most in life. In the face of cruel persecution, what they imagined, and thereby expected, held them steadfast. They believed in God, God as they knew God in Jesus Christ. That belief envisioned a reality with God in charge despite all appearances to the contrary.

Newer understanding of the mind-body relationship makes credible such serenity in the face of adversity. Empirical investigations are replacing "pious hope" in understanding the mechanisms involved in healing (Rossi 1986, 104). Psychiatrist Carl Jung referred to the emotional intensity which remedies reduced adaptability as the transcendent function in which conscious and unconscious information collaborate (Rossi 1986, 85-86). The new brain and the old brain work together in remarkable ways.

Mind-Body Relationship

Since the 1960s, information theory has provided a conceptual base for defining biological brain and psychological mind in a common language (Rossi 1986, 175). That base is useful in understanding how all processes -- biological and mental -- consist in the change and transformation of information. Mental information and biological information are convertible to each other without losing the basic form of the information. We can view the brain, then, as made up of a biological system of information -- the old cortex -- and a mental representational or belief system of information -- the neocortex -- which pass information back and forth.

The limbic system, especially regulated by the hypothalamus, serves as the major converter of information between mind and body. Under conditions of relaxation the system converts neural messages into neuroharmonal "messenger molecules" which activate metabolism, growth, activity, and healing by the immune system.

Under conditions of stress the system reverses those processes, retarding metabolism, growth, activity, and well-being.

This deep part of the brain (Rossi 1986, 116) functions in a way which Norman Cousins characterized as "the doctor who resides within" (quoted by Rossi 1986, 15) and which Augustine identified as "the inner Physician" (Augustine [1955], Bk.X, 203). Somatic information becomes semantic information (Rossi 1986, 22, 24). Belief converts mental information into physical behavior which translates the information into bodily processes.

Thus right hemisphere trust elicits parasympathetic relaxation which results in biochemical healing (Rossi 1986, 23). Such is the explanation of what is commonly known as "the placebo response." The healing potential of the placebo response consists of constructive suggestion, anxiety reduction, and positive expectancy aroused by our belief system, "mediated by the . . . right cerebral hemisphere" (Rossi 1986, 18).

Because a sense of the whole, or God, exceeded a sense of the parts, or the persecutors, we can speculate about what happened in the Christian martyrs. There must have been "an affective discharge via the right-brain-limbic connection . . . an experience [of numinosity or religious awe] during which the connotation of what [was] perceived vastly exceed[ed] the denotation" (d'Aquili 1986, 157). They must have experienced a realistic reality in that the aggressive power of the amygdala -- survival of the self at the expense of others -- was present, but finally they exhibited a hope-filled reality in that the immediate realism was subordinate to the affiliative power of the septum -- continuity of the human species at the expense of self.

The integration of the two hemispheres occurs only at the nonconscious level of the limbic system and expresses itself in consciousness only by means of symbolic representation (d'Aquili 1986; Winson [1985] 1986). As the major system of mind-body communication, the autonomic nervous systems of the martyrs had to have functioned in a way to produce a sense of well-being, a healing of heart and mind in the power of belief in a "new" reality here-and-now.

Sometimes, however, imagination runs wild. We imagine the worst instead of the best, devastation rather than possibility. We "overread" and therefore "overinterpret" the meaning of a situation. We fill the open psychic space with fear and dread. In the language of general systems theory, the limbic system "oscillates" or "runs away." This refers to a pathological reaction in which the self-regulating processes break down. The system destabilizes and disintegrates (Hampden-Turner 1981, 84). In those moments the surge of adrenalin, the arousal of the sympathetic nervous system, takes over and we live in a state of emergency.

A future with hope -- eschatological expectancy -- turns into an impending disaster -- an apocalyptic catastrophe. Possibilities of positive change are not only inconceivable -- a left brain activity -- but even more they are unimaginable -- a right brain activity. The survival vigilance of the amygdala inhibits the cooperative responsiveness of the septum. Physical tension, with its accompanying anxiety, makes relaxation, with its accompanying excitement, impossible. The result is a universe perceived to be -- believed to be -- limiting and limited. Nothing is for us; everything is against us. Natural challenge has been transformed into unavoidable threat.

Since language is never one dimensional, our language-making ability is a resource in re-construing a limiting interpretation. Everyday language is capable of multiple meanings -- metaphorical, figurative, suggestive (Watzlawick 1978). Images generate ideas and ideas have their origin in images. The imaginative mind frees us from the constrictions of the past in the power of "a new heaven and a new earth" (Revelation 21:1), a possibility which is capable of transforming old reality into new reality.

By virtue of its pattern making activity, the right brain is holistic. Values embrace both the very personal and the genuinely communal. Mosaics of meaning continually generate what is intrinsically satisfying. We can approach problems by imaging the future as already present as a working reality. We can create -- and re-create -- "what is" in accordance with what we imagine to be "really real." We can trust that because God is present in all things and in all ways, everything and every way work together for the well-being of all (Romans 8:28).

Whole Brain Integration: Caring for the World

I have described four aspects of the brain -- the naming and analyzing of left hemisphere proclamation and the immersed and imaginative processes of right hemisphere manifestation (Table 6). To stop here, however, obscures their motivating source and their cognitive clarity. In fact, to stop with right and left brain belief would be like cutting our heads off and living without bodies. It would leave us in a disembodied state of being, a view which the church has regarded as a distortion of genuine faith. We embody our faith; therefore, the question becomes: what do our bodies contribute to belief?

We can identify which half of the brain -- left or the right -- and which part of the brain -- sensory input or motor output -- are primary in any particular situation. That activity, however, comes as a result of decisions made below consciousness in the limbic system -- the old mammalian brain, the emotional mind, or what we ordinarily think of as "the body." When I refer to "the brain," I include what is ordinarily thought of as "the body." In the more conventional metaphor by which we live that means our "heart," the source of our deepest feeling of relatedness to others and to the world.

We are learning that the neocortex, with its different ways of handling information, approaches problems either by a rational explanation or a relational responsiveness. Whether we come at a situation analytically or experientially depends upon an emotional choice as to how best to handle what we assume to be the truth of

TABLE 6 BELIEF PATTERNS ORGANIZED BY BRAIN PROCESSES

Hemisphere Strategy	Left Brain Step-by-Step	Right Brain All-at-Once
Belief Pattern	proclaming redemption saving the world	manifesting creation savoring the world
biblical ideas:	Exodus prophetic Word-event the cross future eschatology	Easter priestly Image-event incarnation/resurrection realized eschatology
theological ideas:	wrath judgment dogmatic theology not-yet realized Protestant Principle	love mercy apologetic theology always-already realized Catholic Substance
philosophical ideas:	logos Thomistic cosmology doctrine verbal	eros Augustinian ontology experience preverbal
focus of intention:	history politics ethics loyal obedience	metaphysics mysticism aesthetics trusting dependence
dominant sensory system used:	auditory hearing	visual seeing & sensing feeling

The above strategy patterns are derived from decisions
at the limbic level of activity about   faithful adaptation
to the immediate context or environment.

Belief Pattern	Prophetic Mysticism/Prophetic Action caring for the world	
focus of intention	oppression and liberation	
forms of oppression:	principalities & powers	suffering
forms of theology:	political protest	liberation promise
limbic systems:	amygdala arousal	septum relaxation
behavior focus:	preserve the self	continue the species nurture others
hemisphere strategy		collaboration evaluation

the situation. Conscious activity implements nonconscious perception. It is "out of the heart" that we determine the issues of life.

Let me explain. The fibers of the core brain -- the bridge between the instincts of the reptilian brain and the cognition of the new brain -- connect with every region of the cerebral hemispheres as well as with all the sensory and motor fibers of the brain stem. This core system is proving to be far more differentiated than had previously been supposed (Trevarthen 1986, 191). It is at the level of the old brain -- the emotional mind -- that we select the strategies we regard as best for the survival of the self, for the continuity of the species, and for the nurturing of one another.

Here is the motivational source for our acting rationally in the world in terms of proclamation and acting relationally in terms of manifestation. In the core brain, drawing as it does upon the other two brains, we find what we may speak of in religious language as the world-integrating process of prophetic mysticism. The conventional patterns of belief are primarily conscious interpretations of more primary patterns of emotion.

Integrated activity depends upon higher cortical processing as well as limbic activity. A bottom-up perspective, that is moving from a lower level of organization to a higher level, gives us the components of motivation. In short, the heart effects the head. A top-down perspective, that is moving from a higher level of organization to a lower level, provides us with the components of evaluation. In effect, the head rules the heart (Skinner 1987).

An assessment of how well the strategies work depends on the contribution of both hemispheres, in fact, on all parts of the brain. That collaboration is more than simply the contribution of each hemisphere. It depends upon the maturation of the corpus callosum, the connecting fiber track which lets each side know what the other side knows.

The corpus callosum matures neurologically around the age of twelve. Only then are the activation levels of the two halves equal-ized and coordinated (Levy 1985b, 11-13). Only then can our conscious mind and our nonconscious brain come together in a fully integrating and genuinely fulfilling harmony. Only then can we experience the "aha" of insightful discovery or the "awe" of inspired revelation. Only then can what we feel with our bodies and what we think with our minds be one and the same (Gendlin 1979). Only then are we wholly one, reality with integrity, made in the image of the really real. Only then do we breathe a deep sigh of contentment, knowing that we know all-together, through and through. Only then is life really right.

As the corpus callosum matures, we develop a conscious idea of the self and of our influence on others. With that consciousness two sets of ideas appear: (1) good and bad as these relate to our social behavior, and (2) good and bad as these relate to a universal ideal of what constitutes a person and what goes into a relationship. The "ideal" reflects the new brain transforming information from the old brain into a mental representation, which information, in turn, the new brain has to transform back into old brain process. In effect, here is the grandeur and misery of *homo sapiens*: we must know consciously in our cerebral cortex what we know nonconsciously in our old brain, and we must choose to act in accordance with that knowledge of optimal evolutionary adaptation.

From a neuropsychological viewpoint psychiatrist Eugene d'Aquili has proposed what to me is the most plausible conjecture linking brain process with belief practice. It is

> a model integrating recent split-brain research with W.R. Hess' ergotropic [energy expanding] and trophotropic [energy conserving] model of neural tuning in order to explain the emotional resolution of [polar] opposites presented in myth [such as light and dark, good and evil] which has been integrated into ceremonial ritual . . . the repetitive aspects of ceremonial ritual, whether they be solemn movement,

dance, chanting, drum-beating, and so on, drive the er-
gotropic-dominant hemisphere system to the point of
third stage autonomic tuning. Thus, at nodal points
during ceremonial ritual, third stage autonomic tuning
results in spillover from the ergotropic-major hemisphere system to the trophotropic-minor hemisphere
system, so that both systems fire maximally. . . . The
simultaneous firing of both systems creates a brief
"oceanic" sense of ineffable unity, during which the logical opposites of myth elements are briefly but powerfully united (d'Aquili 1986, 141-142).

When we are tired or stressed or strained, our mental capacity slips
back into earlier stages of development. We regress, as the saying
has it. We experience one part taking over from another part in
competitive or uncoordinated frustration. We act in ways which
fail to take into account important information, either from the
situation in which we find ourselves or from our own internal
processes.

It is at the level of the new brain or the conscious mind that we
evaluate how appropriate a strategy is. Only here do we properly
come together -- body and soul, brain and mind, self and setting.
Only in the integration of all three minds do world-transformation
and world-affirmation find integrity in fulfillment and fulfillment
with integrity. In the maturity of the whole brain, I suggest, we
find the locus of the world-fulfilling activity of prophetic action.
We are responsible for caring for the world with which we have
been graced.

In the last quarter of a century the theological world has erupted,
blossomed, proliferated -- characterize it as we do -- with a third
pattern of belief (Tracy 1981, 390-404). The phenomenon goes by
various labels: liberation theology, third world theology, feminist
theology, black theology, political theology, Latin American theology (Chopp 1986), third-eye theology (Song 1979), water-buffalo
theology (Koyama 1976, among many). The trajectory or family

resemblance, to use Tracy's designation, combines what is real in prophetic mysticism with what is right in prophetic action. In each of these newer theologies we find a radical immersion in specific contexts, responsibility rooted in personal and communal relationships, an integration of right acting with real participating, an indivisible union of human effort with divine power. Means are ends and ends are means.

We are witnessing a basic shift in the locus of the holy. Traditionally people have been oriented to saving or savoring -- worldtransformation, with its proclamation of redemption in a left brain strategy, or to world-affirmation, with its manifestation of creation in a right brain strategy. Today the locus of reality is neither in a specific place, such as Jerusalem or the altar on which Christ was sacrificed as symbolized by the thrusting spire of Chartres Cathedral, nor in most any place as symbolized by the embracing dome of St. Sophia. Instead, the locus of the holy is to be found in concrete historical contexts of human oppression which call for human liberation. The Center organizes what matters to genuine humanity. If we are centered, we can find our way.

Perhaps the phenomenon of liberation theologies represents a return to the experience of the early Christian community. For that community, Christ was a recent and vivid memory. God had raised up the crucified Jesus, making him "both Lord and Christ" (Acts 2:32-36). Out of "old" reality came a "new" reality -- unexpected, life transforming, breaking down "the dividing wall of hostility" between insiders and outsiders and reconciling all in one human family, "the household of God" (Ephesians 2:11-22). Maybe we are discovering ourselves directed toward the creation of a "new heaven and a new earth" in the here-and-now of every particular people in every particular culture in no less a manner than our early Christian ancestors. Those people who turn the world upside down appear everywhere (Acts 17:6b).

The prophetic orientiation focuses on how people act more than on what people say. Each concrete situation calls into question the dominant cultural rationale which justifies structures of inequality -- racism, sexism, classism, ethnocentricism. Cultural development is called into account for its violation of God's created order. Responsible care for the whole created world matters more than anything else.

Brain mechanisms make understandable that shift in belief from saving and savoring to caring.

Cultural information and genetic information combine in conformity to the requirements of the cosmos. The genetic code is not ultimate nor are cultural codes ultimate. Rather, they are derived from and reflections of the ultimate reality of all living systems. Genotypes and culture types are components in which their values are for the whole system and not for any particular part of the system. Failure to function inclusively -- on behalf of all, family, friend, neighbor and enemy alike -- guarantees the demise of every power elite.

The limbic system's transaction between the immediate situation and long term evolutionary adaptation is proving more fundamental to life than the new brain's styles and strategies. We are discovering the primacy of the reptilian brain's instinctual behavior which involves territoriality -- a place of one's own as well as the place of one's species. Ritual, protocol, home territory, native land -- these reveal our groundedness, literally and figuratively. We are discerning the mediation of the mammalian brain's emotional guidance which transforms neural messages into recognizable meaning. Relating, surviving and cooperating, communicating and caring, imaging experience for the sake of integrating that experience into ongoing memory -- these establish our world, literally and symbolically.

Two biblical events become more intelligible in view of the primacy of the limbic process. One comes from the Old Testament and the other from the New Testament. Each can be read in terms of the working brain.

Moses reacted violently when he came upon an Egyptian beating a Hebrew (Exodus 2:11-15). He killed the Egyptian only to discover the crime was noticed. In that moment he fled from his life of privilege, becoming a fugitive from justice.

In the wilderness he found himself face to face with God. The transcendent dimension -- the cosmic connection -- broke through into consciousness. The historical dimension -- the cultural context -- became the arena of ultimate reality. In terms of the brain analogy, the limbic components of survival of self, preservation of species, care of others, and assimilation of new experience with previous experience took on communicable form. The new brain heard the old brain reminding it of its responsibility:

> And Moses hid his face, for he was afraid to look at God. Then the Lord said, "I have seen the affliction of my people who are in Egypt, and have neard their cry because of their taskmasters; I know their sufferings, and I have come down to deliver them. . . . Come, I will send you to Pharaoh that you may bring forth my people . . . out of Egypt" (Exodus 3: 6-10 RSV).

At the threshold of his ministry Jesus, like Moses, found himself in the wilderness. There he wrestled with what it meant to be who he was and what he was to be about. The subcortical reality of relatedness to the really right found its way into the cortical reality of self-consciousness. The result was an empowering by the Spirit. Like Moses he too returned to his immediate context and declared the truth of what life is about (Luke 4:1-17).

> The Spirit of the Lord is upon me, because [God] has anointed me to preach good news to the poor. [God] has sent me to proclaim release to the captives and recovering of sight to the blind, to set at liberty those who are oppressed, to proclaim the acceptable year of the Lord (Luke 4:18-19 RSV).

Each of these events occurred in an historical context, which means in a cultural situation. Belief showed itself in action rather than in thought, though thinking was not absent. The way the brain works helps make that contextualization understandable.

Theologies of proclamation and manifestation appear at the cerebral level reflecting left and right brain cognition. These cortical expressions, however, have their motivational source in the subcortical level of the emotional mind. At that level we find ourselves in a reciprocal relationship with both the culture into which we are born and the environment of which we are an expression. Our brain works to relate what we do with where we are in a way that makes sense rationally. In other words, our actions reflect evolutionary adaptability, or in theological language, conformance to the will of God.

The limitation of the belief pattern of prophetic action comes when the context is restricted to parochial interests as against more universal interests. We restrict what we do to the service of those who are like us and those whom we like. There is no room for the stranger and the enemy. Yet it is precisely in the face of the stranger (Exodus 22:21; 23:9; Leviticus 19:33) and the face of the enemy (Matthew 5:43-48) that we find our truest and fullest human meaning. God is the inclusive reality. To the extent that belief limits life, God selects against exclusiveness.

I connect the old brain and belief this way: in prophetic action promised liberation arises from the reciprocal relationship between energy expansion and energy conservation. Concern for truth -- a left brain vigilance motivated by sympathetic tension and evaluated by the frontal lobes with information from both hemispheres -- is integrated with fidelity to the context -- a right brain responsiveness reflective of parasympathetic relaxation. Prophetic mysticism found in the old brain binds us to our evolutionary niche. We experience an integration with the whole created order. Furthermore and finally, prophetic action, which originates in the new brain, directs us to responsible care which fulfills our destiny in the world.

Quite simply, we do what we do because of where we are.

NOTES

1. The literature is extensive. Among the easily available and better materials see: Edwards (1979; 1986); Perkins (1981); Barbara Brown (1973); Chall and Mirsh (1978); Houston (1982); Linda V. Williams (1983); Wonder and Donovan (1984); Buzan (1985); Durka and Smith (1979).

2. New Testament scholar and translator Donald S. Deer has kindly made me aware of this issue of translating "kardia" as mind. In the standard Greek-English lexicon of the New Testament, "kardia" refers to "the faculty of thought, of the thoughts themselves, of understanding, as the organ of natural and spiritual enlightenment" (Arndt et al [1957] 1979, 403). In this area "kardia" may often be translated "mind." The following passages can be, and have been, so translated: Matthew 9.4; 13.15a,b; 15.19; 24.28; Mark 2.6,8; 3.5; *6.52; 7.21; *8.17; 11.23; Luke *2.19,35, 51; 3.15; 5.22; 9.47; 12.45; 24.25,38; John *12.40a,b; Acts 7.23; 16.14; 28,27a,b; Romans 1.21; 10.6; 16.18; 1 Corinthians 2.9; 2 Corinthians 3.15; 4.6; Ephesians 1.18; 4.18; 1 John 1.26; 2 Peter 1,19; Revelation 18.7. *Cf. Twentieth Century, Goodspeed, New English Bible, and Good News Bible -- which each translates these verses as indicated; King James Version, New American Standard Bible, Revised Standard Version, and New International Version, according to Deer, mistranslate these verses.

3. The left brain and right brain dimensions of belief are speculative. Pierce (1986) verified and measured these cognitive dimensions empirically, which adds support for my impressionistic mapping. The three dimensions which accounted for 92 percent of the variance were: Cost of Discipleship versus Blessing of God; In-

strumental versus Relational-Symbolic; and Human Efforts versus Divine Power. The first pole in each dimension correlated with my hypothesized left brain redemption oriented belief pattern, while the second pole in each dimension correlated with my hypothesized right brain creation oriented belief pattern. I elaborate these dimensions in the chapter on gender issues. (For an earlier and more detailed description of the typology of believing mind-states, see Ashbrook 1984b; 1984c.) Brain Technologies Corporation has developed The Brain Map for what it calls "Neuropreneuring," or "the principles and practices of self-directed change," particularly as these relate to business and marriage. Although it is not yet verified empirically, it is a remarkably useful instrument for individuals and/or groups in encouraging responsibility, making lost or distorted information available, and developing constructive and creative approaches to working relationships.

CHAPTER NINE

OUR SENSORY SYSTEMS AS LANGUAGE

If people see with their eyes,
and hear with their ears,
and understand with their hearts,
[then they will] turn and be healed.
(Isaiah 6:10 RSV)

They heard something --
like the rush of a mighty wind;
They saw something --
like tongues of fire;
they felt something --
being filled with the Holy Spirit.
(Acts 2:1-4)

What people take as metaphor is literally true.

We lose a quality of life when we lose our sensory system or it becomes inactive. But from birth and early childhood the sensory system was all we had to understand the world. Gradually we developed language and that informed us on a different level. We lost sensory perception and learning in the exchange. The issue is to regain the sensory system or give it its crucial place. Emphasis on right brain functioning may be a tool by which this might be done.

The Bible calls us to account for our lack of sensory processing. Eyes that do not see, ears that do not hear, hearts that do not feel -- cut off from God and one another through ignorance and insensitivity. That describes the human condition (Psalm 135:15-18; Isaiah 6:10; Matthew 13:14-16; John 12:40; Ephesians 4:18). Like Nasrudin's donkeys, our senses have been with us always, right in front of us, in truth, part of our very existence, from the beginning, and yet we have missed the subtlety of the obvious.

The senses are basic to life, basic to believing, basic to our being the genuinely human beings God means us to be. We have tended to disembody faith, separate the spiritual from the physical, genuine life from sensory processing -- seeing, hearing, and feeling, not to mention smelling, tasting, and touching. We come closest to the power of these processes in complaints about people being "blind" to reality, "deaf" to the truth, or "insensitive" to suffering.

Few have shifted from the sensory capacity as a symbolic interpretation of human experience to the sensory processes as actual mechanisms of meaning and for meaning. In the last dozen years, however, neurolinguistic programming (NLP) has achieved wide acceptance among professional counselors and psychotherapists by mapping the sensory systems for more effective communication (Bandler and Grinder 1975; Grinder and Bandler 1976). NLP identifies how people construct their individual worlds based upon how they access and process sensory information, most especially the auditory, kinesthetic and visual representational systems.

These representational systems (1) constitute maps or models of reality, (2) which we construct on the basis of transforming raw sensory stimuli into re-presentations of that data, (3) which we then use as representations of the world in which we live, and (4) on the basis of which we act in that world as we have constructed it. With the knowledge accumulating in the cognitive and neurological sciences we now can use sensory metaphors as explicit means to fuller human meaning.

For me the connection between brain and belief came in a workshop with black pastors serving inner city churches.

I was telling them about neurolinguistic processing and the way some people prefer the visual system, others the auditory system, and still others the kinesthetic system. I put the issue colloquially by saying that some of us are "eye" people, others "ear" people, and most of us "visceral" or "gut" people. At that point the Rev. Samuel Adams of Syracuse, New York, burst out: "You're talking about Pentecost: they *saw* something; they *heard* something; they *felt* something (Acts 2:1-4)!" He had connected Bible and brain. Once we realized the truth of that connection we returned to the Bible, to our patterns of belief and to our own everyday lives with renewed minds. Rather dramatically we woke up, came to our senses as happened to the Prodigal Son (cf. Luke 15:17), literally seeing the reality of "donkeys" in our lives for the first time.

The subtle had become obvious. We no longer were cut off from reality through "ignorance and insensitivity" (Ephesians 4:18). The truth of our seeing, hearing and feeling was apparent everywhere.

Experiencing The Subtle

In Chapter Three I suggested several exercises which made it possible for you to experience something of the different processes in the two hemispheres. You became aware of the fact that people fold their hands differently. You sensed that each side of your body carries different responses for different qualities of experience. You found you used different kinds of words to describe yourself depending upon which hand you used to write them. Each of these exercises reflects the crossed structure of our nervous system so that the left hemisphere controls the right side of the body and the right hemisphere controls the left side of the body. The discussion of sensory systems takes us further into that cross over processing.

Take a moment to try the following exercises (Bandler and Grinder 1979, 18-27):

How many windows are there in the place where you live?

How many traffic lights are there between your home and where you do your grocery shopping?

What clothes will you wear to the next party you attend?

If you had a choice between going to a concert, a baseball game or a museum, how would you decide?

Were you aware of what went on inside you in response to each question? If not, go back over the questions and direct your attention to the experience of finding answers. By attending to what goes on inside as we process different tasks we become aware of physical shifts in ourselves. The shifts in attention may be slight but with continuing awareness we can become more conscious of the shifts.

As an aid in identifying those shifts in attention, think back on your experience of what your eyes did as you tried to answer each question. Which questions were your eyes turning toward your left; which questions were your eyes turning toward your right; which questions were your eyes shifting back and forth between your left and your right sides?

Our eyes are controlled by the opposite hemisphere just as our hands and the sides of our body are. For most right-handed people when their eyes turn toward their left it is their right brain which is taking the lead in accessing information needed for the task. Similarly when their eyes turn toward their right it is their left brain which is taking the lead in accessing information needed for the task. We can infer that left-turning eyes indicate a right brain process of intouch imaginative responsiveness or, more simply, finding "what is," primarily matters involving space and past experience. Right-turning eyes indicate a left brain process of intentional analytical vigilance or, actually, searching for "what might be," primarily matters involving time and future possibilities.

The nature of the task usually determines which hemisphere takes the lead in processing information (Edwards 1979, 42-43). Two factors, however, influence the question of control. One includes a decision as to which brain can get the job done fastest; the other a decision as to which brain is more invested in the task. In short, speed and motivation (Levy and Trevarthen 1976).

Generally, the left brain tends to be the more assertive of the two because of its interpretive structuring of a rationale for what it observes, as with the split brain patient who claimed his left hand selected the shovel in order to clean out the chicken shed (despite the fact the right brain was acting on the basis of having seen a snow scene). Our brains are wired to stabilize the environment, to simplify complexity in terms of assumptions about "reality" and the way we organize information (Ornstein [1972, 1977] 1986, 21-38). That stability comes as we give names to stimuli, thereby creating discrete objects with clear boundaries. Art teacher Betty Edwards provides detailed instructions to help people experience a shift from the left mode of processing to the right mode (Edwards 1979, 45-59). Basically, the instructions require engaging in activities which "remain nameless" since "naming" is a left brain competence.

I want to caution against too much generalization at this point. As I have indicated in various places, our individual brains are as unique as our fingerprints. Any particular person will manifest patterns uniquely their own and so distinctly different from much of the rest of the population. For left-handers and about 20% of right handers who have a mixed dominance such as writing with the right hand and lighting a match with the left (Goleman 1985), inferences about the direction of their eye turning, the activation of the opposite hemisphere in finding "what is" by the right brain or creating "what might be" by the left brain is uncertain. Not only do we each have our own consistencies but we each also have our own inconsistencies.

Keeping those qualifications in mind, I make three assumptions about how we use our brain:

> (1) under ordinary circumstances we tend to value and rely upon preferred (Grinder and Bandler 1976, 9-15) and familiar responses. That means we draw upon a

primary sensory system and use only part of the cortical capacity;

(2) under inspiring conditions we have a wider range of responses available. That leads to our drawing upon every sensory system and every part of the cortex in an optimally adaptive combination of tension and relaxation in the service of the self in its contribution to the continuity of the species; and

(3) under anxious or stressful circumstances we fall back upon the most used and so more valued representational processing. The result is that we draw upon a single sensory system and a single part of the cortex, those patterns of our lives which are the most ingrained and the most automatic in coping with the survival of the self. The other systems either process information in a way which is incongruent and at odds with that system or else fuzzy and so not easily understandable (Grinder and Bandler 1976, 27-96, 97-122).

In brief, most of the time we rely upon a limited amount of sensory information; occasionally we utilize more information; under pressure we clutch at limiting information, limiting in that we fail to take in information necessary for optimal adaptation. We simply do not act in our own best interest -- even though we think we are.

What is subtle in experience seems complicated to understand. Yet in discerning the subtle we discover the obvious.

Discovering The Obvious

I once heard an argument between the president of an educational institution and his director of public relations. The president asked the director what he thought of a certain problem. The director responded by reporting how he felt about it. After several such exchanges the president exploded in frustration: "I don't care what you 'feel,' I want to know what you 'think'!" The exchange sounded like many I had heard between chairmen of Boards of Trustees and their pastors.

Looking back to that impasse, I now understand that the director of public relations was organizing information in terms of his kinesthetic sensory system, that is "feeling." In contrast, the president was organizing information in terms of his auditory sensory system, that is "thinking." Neither realized the other came at life through different ways of processing information. They assumed they were referring to the same reality when in fact they were functioning on the basis of different realities.

Neurolinguistic programming assumes a connection between sensory processing and verbal communication. More specifically, it describes how the ways people talk reveal their models of the world in which they live. Language reflects our maps of the world.

That clue to the connection between sensing and saying lies specifically with the verbs, adjectives, and adverbs -- the predicates -- we use to describe experience (Grinder and Bandler 1976, 9-12). The president used "think," which is an auditory word; the director used "feel," which is a visceral word; and I used "looking," which is a visual word. These words reflect our unconscious choices and preferences about the best way to represent and communicate what we know.

My native language is English. Almost everyone I know speaks English, though I have contact with people whose native languages are Korean, French, German, Chinese, among others. These languages are the conventional forms in which we think and with which we communicate. Whether we share conventional speech and native language, we all draw upon a more basic grammatical form. In that more basic form language consists of map-making. We transform raw sensory input into organized usable output. We re-present experience in some more organized way.

Maps orient us to what matters (Bandler and Grinder 1975). In so doing they distort the sensation of "what is" in order to convey an idea of the experience of "what is there." They delete information, allowing us to grasp that information essential for our own purposes. They generalize from specific parts of the territory to convey a sense of the terrain as a whole. Obviously a map is not the territory, even though the territory requires a map if it is to be viewed in its entirety.

Accordingly, we all use three primary language maps to re-present and organize experience:

> the language of the ear, which is an auditory map, discernible by the prevalence of such words as listen, think, hear, discuss, detail, say;

> the language of the eye, which is a visual map, discernible by the prevalence of such words as see, focus, picture, perspective, look, show; and

> the language of the body, which is a visceral map or kinesthetic map, discernible by the prevalence of such words as feel, touch, grasp, handle, pressure, sense.

There also are the minor language maps of the nose, which is a smelling or olfactory map, and of the tongue, which is a tasting or gustatory map. These maps are our systems of input designed to take in and re-present "reality." The more maps we use the more territory we have available for our conscious purposes. The fewer maps we use the less territory we have available for our use.

As an aid to keeping these different maps in mind I think of ear language as akin to German. German seems complicated and abstract, just as auditory processing has an abstracting quality to it. I think of eye language as akin to Chinese. Chinese seems pictorial and tangible, just as visual processing has a perceptual quality to it. And I think of visceral language as akin to Swahili. Swahili seems personal and physical, just as kinesthetic processing has a sensing quality to it.

Like Nasrudin's donkeys neurolinguistic programming is helping us discover the obvious. We talk in a conventional language while we think in more primary languages. However, because our sensory systems cross over from one side of the body and are processed by the brain on the other side, these primary languages of ear, eye and body represent experience in contrasting ways.

Each brain uses these languages in a different way -- as we would infer from their different styles of functioning.

Major Sensory Systems

Consider the different way each hemisphere uses sensory information (Kolb and Whishaw [1980] 1985, 186-204, 339-343). Stimuli are initially coded, combined, and finally re-presented in the tertiary forms of which we are consciously aware. Each step beyond the primary sensory cortex involves activity at higher levels of organization which thereby transforms received sensations into active perceptions. The same sensory stimulation can result in totally different perceptions, especially as these are affected by the context in which they occur (Kolb and Whishaw [1980] 1985, 202). In short, we are active organisms and not simply passive organisms on which the environment writes its own script.

In visceral or kinesthetic re-presentation, the left hemisphere processes sensations in a refined, deliberate, controlled and stabilizing way. The right hemisphere processes in a sensual way, one that is spontaneous, natural and impressionistic. When these visceral languages combine, our general sensory experience is richly differentiated within a context which is experienced as all-together yet ever-changing.

In auditory re-presentation, the left hemisphere processes sounds as concepts or symbols identified by narrow meanings, publicly understood as in formal dictionary definitions which do not require a person to understand the implicit context necessary to grasp the meaning of idiomatic expressions. It is the right hemisphere which attends to the felt meaning of the language, the broad, suggestive, experientially based connotations of the sounds. As we combine these auditory languages, we hear in a way which is conceptually clear yet intuitively understandable.

Japan presents a special case of these two ways of hearing and thinking, and thereby an example which clarifies the processes.

The Japanese have adopted two types of written language (Bloom, Lazerson, and Hofstadter 1985, 217). One, known as Kana, uses symbols which represent sounds as our alphabet does, in an item-by-item, letter-by-letter approach. The symbols stand for specific combinations of sounds or syllables. The other, known as Kanji, uses symbols in a more pictorial or ideographic way, an all-at-once approach, with the visual form presenting the intended meaning. Each symbol represents an object or an idea in its entirety rather than a sound in its discreteness.

One further aspect of the way the Japanese people process sounds illustrates the difference between left and right brain strategies and the influence of culture on cortical activity. The Japanese have been noted for their fundamentally sentimental love of na-ture. In that area Westerners have been regarded as more rational and logical. Few of us in the West have bothered attending to crickets chirping, for instance. Yet for centuries Japanese poets have contemplated crickets chirping. In modern Japanese hotels the radio gently wakens the visitor with sounds of crickets and birds. Images of cool autumn evenings float through the air be-cause of the sounds.

Tsunoda Tadabu, noted audiolgist at the Tokyo Medical Dental College, wondered whether such contrasts could reflect differen-ces in the way people process sounds (The East 1975). He com-pared 92 Japanese and 12 Westerners as to which hemisphere took the lead in response to the following: pure vowels in their own language, the crying and humming of human voices, and the sounds of insects and animals. Westerners processed these with the left ear and the right hemisphere, which means they did not give the sounds an interpretive label which objectified them. Japanese, however, processed these sounds with their right ear and left hemisphere, which suggests that they heard the sounds as verbal expressions and therefore as symbolic language. Only the sounds of consonants, orchestral music, calculations and machine noises were heard by both groups in the right hemisphere.

In visual re-presentation, the left hemisphere sees in an objective, permanent, abstract way by attaching a label to a perception. Because of its inability to name what it sees, the right hemisphere sees more in terms of impressions, appearances, and the imaginative (see Edwards 1979). As with the other two major systems, when these two processes are combined we represent what is in its immediacy -- impressionistically and imaginatively.

Predicates do help us discover the obvious. Ear words imply auditory representations of reality; eye words imply visual representations of reality; and body words imply kinesthetic representations of reality. Beyond the major sensory maps, however, we also need to attend to and identify the way in which people use those maps. The hemisphere which takes the lead in dealing with the world influences the way the sensory information is organized, and the way the information is organized reflects the strategy which we choose for dealing with what matters most in the immediate situation.

In brief the left brain creates ordinary reality. The strategy derives from an emotional decision which calls for sympathetic arousal and vigilance. From what it observes it explains everything in a way which is reasonable in its own universe of meaning. It analyzes sounds conceptually. It refines sensations into separate systems and in terms of sequences which it can make conscious. It simplifies sights into objects. Whether the information comes from the auditory (Bever, Hurtig, and Handel 1976), visual (Oscar-Berman, Blumstein, and DeCusa 1976), or tactile (Kolb and Whishaw [1980] 1985, 342-343) system, therefore, everything takes on a standardized form (see Table 3).

The right brain responds to an ever-changing scene from the inside (Mountcastle 1976, 40). This strategy reflects an emotional decision which calls for parasympathetic relaxation and responsiveness to a mosaic of meaning in its entirety. Without a fixed point of reference it experiences everything in ways which are impressionistic and associated. It hears sounds as intonations, feeling (Milner 1962, 187-188), and melody (Kimura 1964). It combines sensations into flowing patterns. It sees visions and dreams dreams (see Table 4).

Having begun to experience the subtle and discover the obvious, we can begin to apply knowledge of sensory processing and representational schema to how we get along in the world -- with ourselves and with others. We get cut off from God and one another, as the writer to the Ephesians has indicated (4:18), through ignorance and insensitivity. To reverse those factors then would offer the possibility of renewed life. Knowledge and sensitivity -- these are clues to being renewed and transformed.

I now examine, in turn, the features of disturbed processing, deficient processing, and whole or holy processing. Each has its biblical correlate, each its pattern of belief, and each its recovery of more adequate functioning.

Body Vs. Mind: Disturbed Processing

Recall St. Paul's vivid description of his "body" battling what his "reason dictates" (Romans 7:23). Little wonder, then, that disturbed processing shows itself in dramatic ways. In normal development researchers assume that cerebral dominance decreases. Increasingly the two hemispheres and the two cognitive styles balance each other, that is, they are complementary and mutually enhancing (Kershner 1985). However, in disturbed development the two styles compete with each other for cerebral dominance. One side struggles with the other side as to which cognitive strategy will take the lead. Input from one sensory system overrides and negates input from other sensory systems. As Jesus pointed out, that which is divided against itself cannot stand (Matthew 12:25).

Right brain outburst clashes with left brain control. Each half is equally powerful. The struggle paralyzes action. Neither half can take the millisecond lead required for integrated response. Similarly, when one strategy preempts the process, the rejected information does not disappear. Instead it works surreptitiously and subversively, undermining and disrupting what we do.

These patterns of competing processes are as true of cultures as they are of individuals. What goes on in the lives of the psychic microcosm reflects what goes on in the culture (TenHouten 1985). Then, from a theological perspective, people experience and perceive in the ontological macrocosm a war between the forces of light and the forces of darkness.

An experience of an eight-year-old boy in play therapy illustrates disturbed processing (Halpern 1963, 15-17). The resolution of the disturbance suggests steps we can take toward reestablishing a more functional balance. He had been referred for treatment because of disruptive behavior at home and in school.

> The youngster had a puppet character named "Noodlehand." Noodlehand would politely say "hello," and then promptly bite people on the nose or chop them up and make them eat bees and spiders. He was a thoroughly obnoxious character.

> After a few months of therapy a new puppet character appeared named "Superhand." Superhand was powerful. He hated evil and evildoers, but because he lived in "Outer Space," he usually was not around when Noodlehand acted up. When he did show up, he smacked and pushed Noodlehand in order to make him behave.

> The two characters increasingly tangled with each other. After a particularly ferocious battle the therapist asked

the boy, "Whom do you want to win: Noodlehand or Superhand?"

"I don't know!" the boy replied with agitation. "If Noodlehand wins, everything will be terrible -- I'll be a mean troublemaker and nobody will like me. But if Superhand wins, I'll be the best little boy in the whole United States, and then everyone will step on me and take advantage of me! I don't know! I don't know!"

The therapist and the boy stood for a long time contemplating the irreconcilable characters. Quietly the therapist suggested, "Maybe nobody has to win. Maybe Noodlehand can stay around to keep people from stepping on you, and Superhand can move in from Outer Space so he can be around to keep Noodlehand from getting out of hand." The boy looked at him with a surprised smile.

The next week a new puppet character appeared. It began to make peace efforts between Noodlehand and Superhand. Its name was "Hand-in-Hand"!

Such a reconciliation between Superhand with its abstract, left mind keep-life-in-check strategy and Noodlehand with its concrete, right mind plunge-ahead-no matter-what strategy reveals harmony-in-action. It is more than conscious intention. It reflects the deep reality in which we participate but which we do not create. It arises from an integration of emotions concerned with both survival of the self and cooperation with others. These processes arise below the cerebral cortex at the limbic level, with the coordinated activity of the assertive amygdala and the adaptive septum (MacLean 1977, 159-160). At the same time the resolution is purposive and singleminded, whole brained, by virtue of reflection about more adaptive behavior.

From this example we can specify steps which contribute to more balanced processing (Grinder and Bandler 1976, 27-96):

Step One: The conflicted sides are resorted into separate "realities." What had been all-mixed-together into <u>one</u> bad boy became <u>two</u> puppet characters -- Noodlehand and Superhand. As the conflict was allowed to emerge into fuller consciousness, the task required moving from an all-mixed-together experience into separate-sequential processes. The mismatch of sensory information between Noodlehand's visceral system and Superhand's visual system was reduced.

Step Two: Each "new" process needs to develop its own character more fully. That makes for a coherent self, one style expressed through every sensory system. Noodlehand's outburst could be consistent because it felt outburst; it saw outburst; it talked outburst; it was <u>all</u> outburst. Every sensory system processed outburst. Superhand's order could be consistent because it felt order; it talked order; it saw order; it was <u>all</u> order. Every sensory system processed order. Each part occupied its own space. Each developed its own thoughts, its own feelings, its own fantasies. Each acted in a coordinated and consistent manner.

Step Three: Each "person" is encouraged to express its own part in the drama, in turn, unhindered by its counterpart. The characters are free to be all that they can be: consistently, systematically, even exaggeratedly. Their places are assured; their presence established; their input essential.

Step Four: Eventually, each part must deal with the other part. Isolated and independent activity are eliminated. The polarities are integrated through dialogue between each other. A Noodlehand and a Superhand belong together. So each challenges, questions, opposes, and converses with the other. Questions tumble out: How do we interfere with each other?

How can we use each other? What is the truth we each of possess? Neither character escapes the fact it is a *part* and not the whole. They are intertwined. Trouble for one means trouble for the other. The only way out is to find a way together.

Step Five: Unexpectedly from such an open struggle a synthesis emerges. As the wind blows where it wills, so spiritual singlemindedness emerges in surprising ways (John 3:8). Opposite strategies turn out to be complementary. Hand-in-Hand integrates left mind regularity with right mind spontaneity. Two sides show themselves as one whole: balanced, coordinated, congruent, intentional about what is right and intouch with what is real.

Disturbed experience requires a reconciliation of conflicting processes. The corpus callosum makes such partnership-in-dialogue possible (Levy 1985). Each side lets the other side know what it knows for the sake of the whole. Isaiah provides an image for this direction: "The wolf shall live with the sheep, and the leopard lie down with the kid; the calf and the young lion shall grow up together, and a little child shall·lead them . . ." (Isaiah 11:6-7 NEB). Here then is a new reality -- "to create out of the two a single new humanity . . . thereby making peace . . ." (Ephesians 2:15 NEB).

God acts to create a new time, that is, a rebirth or being born again (John 3:1-21).

With our first birth we lose an original singlemindedness. Consciousness makes for self-consciousness, and self-consciousness makes for separation, and separation generates tension between the self and its world. All this makes for a cognitive complexity which is qualitatively different from other mammals. Manifestations of God thereby appear ambiguous, often in conflict, and always open to mis-representation.

The hermeneutic of proclamation challenges such disturbed processing. It requires each distortion to give an account of itself. It sets right the conditions which make manifest that which has been present always-already. Much of the power of the raging psalmists comes precisely from their antiphonal cries of hurt and hope. Each response is an experienced whole, singleminded and congruent in both its source and its expression. Before God we can rage, reflect and rejoice (Troeger 1980).

Neither Cold Nor Hot: Deficient Processing

If there is too much input in disturbed processing, there is not enough going on in deficient processing. In the Letter to The Church of Laodicea God castigates them for being "neither cold nor hot. Would that you were cold or hot. So, because you are lukewarm, and neither cold not hot, I will spew you out of my mouth" (Revelation 3:15-16 RSV). This is a vivid caricature of deficient processing.

Necessary data are simply unavailable. Without stimuli the spirit atrophes. Such neglect comes as people use only one cognitive style and only one sensory system to engage reality. In these circumstances the other style and the rarely used sensory systems require special attending to. We are to be both cold and hot.

When only the left mind has functioned, more use of the right mind is called for. Initially that means blocking left brain rationality (Watzlawick 1978, 91-126; Edwards 1979, 45-59). Although this kind of approach has been criticized as simplistic and misleading (Harris 1985, 262-267), I am not arguing for processing strategies as specifically correlated with the left and right hemispheres. Instead I am directing attention to various processing possibilities by speaking of the left brain/right brain distinction metaphorically.

Conceptualizations must be de-conceived, that is, transformed from ideas back into images and sensations. In technical language, that is known as de-automatization (Deikman 1969, 30-35). The cognitive structures which "organize, limit, select, and interpret perceptual stimuli" are undone in order to be replaced by "a receptive perceptual mode." For instance, Jeremiah spoke of pulling down and tearing up before building and planting (Jeremiah 1:9-10). We de-structure in order to re-structure. One prevents abstraction by a redirected awareness to immediate experience. A firm conclusion is reframed into an ongoing process.

In short, we shift from left mind expression to right mind experience (Bandler and Grinder 1975, 57-110; Grinder and Bandler 1976, 97-122).

Psychiatrist Milton H. Erickson was a master at such shifts. Because the left mind acts only in terms of what it "thinks," based upon what it "observes," behavior can become sterile. Explanations swallow up experiences. Maps replace the territory. People are neither cold nor hot, only lukewarm, insipid, deficient. So, Erickson engaged people in ways which broke up their self-limiting cycles by generating re-newed experience. Jay Haley (1973, 164-166) describes one such dramatic re-presentation of stimuli.

> A highly educated professional couple came to Erickson because of their inability to conceive and have a child. They had married at age 30, both being excessively prudish and formal.
>
> The husband voiced their predicament: "In my thinking, and that of my wife, we have reached the conclusion that it is more proper that I give voice to our trouble in common and state it succinctly. Our problem is most distressing and destructive of our marriage. Because of our desire for children we have engaged in the marital union with full physiological concomitants each night and morning for procreative purposes. On Sundays and holidays we have engaged in the marital union with full physiological concomitants for procreative purposes as much as four times a day. We have not permitted physi-

cal disability to interfere. As a result of the frustration of our philoprogenitive desires, the marital union has become progressively unpleasant for us, but it has not interfered with our efforts at procreation; but it does distress both of us to discover our increasing impatience with each other. For this reason we are seeking your aid, since other medical aid has failed."

The wife stated her view of the problem in exactly the same abstract and formal manner, only with even more embarrassment.

Erickson told them: "I can correct this for you, but it will involve shock therapy. It will not be electric shock or physical shock but it will be a matter of psychological shock. I will leave you alone in the office for fifteen minutes so that the two of you can exchange views and opinions about your willingness to receive a rather severe psychological shock. At the end of fifteen minutes I will come back into the office and ask your decision and abide by it."

Upon his return, he demanded, "Give me your answer." The man again spoke: "We have discussed the matter both objectively and subjectively, and we have reached the conclusion that we will endure anything that might possibly offer satisfaction for our philoprogenitive desires." The wife concurred.

Erickson explained the psychological shock as a definite strain upon their emotions. "It will be rather simple to administer, but you will both be exceedingly shocked psychologically. I suggest that as you sit there in your chairs, you reach down under the sides of your chairs and hang tightly to the bottom of the chair and listen well to what I say. After I have said it, and as I am administering the shock, I want the two of you to maintain an absolute silence. Within a few minutes you will be able to leave the office and return to your home. I want the two of you to maintain an absolute silence all the way home, and during the silence you will discover a multitude of thoughts rushing through your minds. Upon reaching home, you will maintain silence until after you have entered the house and closed the door. You will then be free! Now hang tightly to the bottom of your chairs, because I am going to give you the psychological shock. It is this: For three long years you have engaged in the marital union with full physiological concomitants for procreative purposes at least twice a day and sometimes as much as four times in twenty-four hours, and you have met with defeat of your philoprogenitive desires. Now why in hell don't you fuck for fun and pray to the devil that she isn't knocked up for at least three months. Now please leave."

Later they told him they had maintained absolute silence during the forty-mile drive home. Many vivid thoughts, feelings, and images raced through each of their minds. Once inside the house with the door shut, according to the husband, "We found we couldn't wait to get to the bedroom. We just dropped to the floor. We didn't engage in the marital union; we had fun." When Erickson talked with them nine months later after a baby girl was born, "formal speech and polysyllabic words and highly proper phrases were no longer necessary."

The "neither cold nor hot" deficiency illustrated in this couple was also apparent in the group to whom Erickson related the case. The audience of practicing psychiatrists, listening to the report, "froze into rigid mobility" at "the utterance of the keyword" "fuck." The residual effects of language inhibitions learned in childhood result in deficiency in sensory processing. The explosion into fuller experience discloses a harmony that links sense to sound and sight. It is more than deliberate intouchness. It reflects the deep emotional reality that informs our entire being (MacLean 1977, 159-160).

From this example we can identify steps which contribute to such fuller processing (Zeig 1980):

Step One: The individual's dominant strategy is respected. We do not destroy people's coping patterns. To sweep out their survival mechanism leaves them vulnerable to disintegration (Luke 11:24-26). In the instance of the couple's rational-auditory strategy, Erickson used their style, their perceptions, and their language. In effect, he met them on their territory.

Step Two: We ask for permission to proceed with a challenge. We do not invade people's privacy. So, like the image of Jesus in the Book of Revelation (3:19-20), we stand at the door of their lives and knock. Erickson laid out conditions for change and insisted on free choice: the couple had to think about the consequences before he proceeded.

Step Three: People's curiosity is aroused. By dragging out details and unfolding a story, we keep people attentive and absorbed. All their senses are activated. They listen more alertly; look more closely; feel more keenly. Since the end remains uncertain, the left mind cannot wrap up the experience with a label. The right mind continues to be responsive to what is still to come, namely, the disclosure of the point of the story. One's mapping systems must process in a trial-and-error way. Because truth is likely to be manifested anywhere, people must attend everywhere. So, the couple could receive new input precisely because their left minds could not function as they had.

Step Four: What is abstract is translated back into the concrete. A "fuck for fun" demolishes a "marital union

with full physiological concomitants." People are shocked into seeing and hearing and sensing all-at-once. For
instance, a legal definition of "who is my neighbor?"
gets transformed into the Parable of The Good Samaritan:
"A man was going down from Jerusalem to Jericho, and
he fell among robbers . . ." a priest . . . [and] a Levite . . .
passed by . . . But a Samaritan . . . had compassion [on
him] . . . which of these three, do you think, proved
neighbor to the man who fell among the robbers?"
(Luke 10:25-37 RSV). Vivid imagery dissolves sterile
concepts.

A variety of possibilities can be tried, depending on the particular
sensory system with which we choose to work.

Deficient processing requires emotional as well as cognitive input.
The level of subsidiary awareness, as Polanyi identified it (Polanyi
1966), opens us to the fuller nuances of reality. The felt-meaning
of experience expresses more than formal conceptualization. A
variety of possibilities can be tried, depending on the particular
sensory systems and style of processing we choose to activate.

In terms of hearing, for instance, auditory mapping can utilize "the
language of change." Such a process involves our talking
metaphorically, poetically, figuratively, parabolically, paradoxically
(Watzlawick 1978; McFague 1975; 1982; Shah [1978] 1981; Kubose
1973). Word studies break up fixed definitions by opening up
nuances of meaning, depending upon the various contexts in which
they are used. Brainstorming generates several solutions to a puzzling problem. By playing with words the familiar can be made
strange and the strange familiar (Gordon 1961, 29-31).

Music especially can engage both processes of step-by-step and all-
at-once. For instance (Rosenfeld 1985), Bach-like music tends to
be rational in its mathematical complexity with logical sequences
of rhythm, melody, and movement; its temporal and elongated
phrasing; its individual solos; and its spiraling. Similarly, though

in contrast, folk-like music tends to be emotional in its variedness with simultaneous chords, harmony, and resolution; its vertical and simultaneous sounds; its communal choruses; and its unifying. From social merrymaking to celebrative worshipping (Werner 1962), music opens us to the music of the spheres. The ineffable of human experience is thereby translated into expressions of meaning and meaningful expressions (Bumbar 1979).

Similarly, visual mapping can utilize images (Arnheim 1972; Feldman 1972; Samuels and Samuels 1975; Somer 1978), fantasies, daydreams, and dreams themselves (Bettleheim 1978; Clift and Clift 1984; Ullman & Zimmerman [1979] 1980). Gestalt exercises in perception -- as the classic view of the young woman or/and the old lady -- loosen single configurations for other possibilities. Microscopic attending to a single leaf or snow flake or scanning the horizon for broad vistas each breaks-up limited and, thereby deficient, perceptions.

Visceral experiencing likewise quickens new and renewed perception. From ritual to dance (d'Aquili and Laughlin 1979), from sensory awakening to relaxation procedures (Feldenkrais 1972; Gendlin 1978), the body again takes the lead in reconnecting with the world around and the world within.

The phenomenology of manifestation provides a belief pattern that goes beyond deficient processing. It directs our attention everywhere and anywhere. The locus of the holy, the realm of the real, only awaits our attending to it to come alive. (Johnston 1981) We shift our focus from "putting out" to allowing ourselves to "take in." Instead of acting like taxi drivers rushing to get a passenger to the airport, we become like little children playing with the daisies or monks meditating in the quiet of places apart.

Holy Processing: Invitation To Reality

Evidence of inadequate and distorted living is all too readily apparent. We have been gifted with eyes and ears and hearts. We have diminished those capacities and thereby diminished the image of God among us and the grandeur of God in the world. "[If people] see with their eyes, and hear with their ears, and understand with their hearts, [then they] will turn and be healed" (Isaiah 6:10 RSV).

The splendor of Pentecost holds before us the possibility of rebirth. Dramatic though that sounds, it is more immediately accessible than we have realized (Biersdorf 1985). Willa Cather put it succinctly in "Death Comes for the Archbishop" (Cather 1971, 50):

> The miracles of the Church seem to me to rest not so much upon faces or voices or healing power coming suddenly near to us from afar of faith, but upon our perceptions being made finer, so that for a moment our eyes can see and ears hear what is there about us always.

When we are intouch with "what is there about us always," then we do indeed sing:

> For the joy of ear and eye,
> For the heart and mind's delight,
> For the mystic harmony
> Linking sense to sound and sight:
> Lord of all, to you we raise
> This our hymn of grateful praise.

CHAPTER TEN

TOWARD A NEW CREATION OF BEING

Now I am revealing new things to you,
things hidden and unknown to you,
created just now, at this very moment,
of these things you have heard nothing until now,
so that you cannot say, "Oh yes, I knew all this."
(Isaiah 48:6-7 JB)

In an intriguing study of the Rorschach projective test of emotional and intellectual functioning, Diane Jonte-Pace (1987) presented protocols of three advanced spiritual masters -- a Hindu Vedantist, Swami Sivanande; an Apache Shaman, Black Eyes; and an enlightened Buddhist "master." Herman Rorschach had discovered that the ambiguous sensory stimuli of his inkblots enabled him to infer and measure the relationship between the structure of their perception and the structure of their personality (see Schachtel 1966). Perceptual responses are evaluated according to two major groupings: location scores which include whole, detail, or small detail responses; and determinant scores which include form, color, movement, or shading. The protocols were decisively different and yet remarkably similar.

They differed in content. Each interpreted the cards in a way which reflected the ultimate concerns of his particular culture: the Swami saw the oneness of everything, the Buddhist the suffering in everything, and Black Eyes the life force in nature and the cycle of seasons. These responses came in an integrated, sequential, and systematic way as each subsumed his individual identity to that of his spiritual and cultural identity. These integrated protocols showed "no universalism of response," which is not surprising in terms of what we know of the shaping of the brain by the impact of culture. Culture provides the means by which we perceive, represent, and interpret experience.

However, the masters were remarkably similar in the way they dealt with the cards -- in their style of response and in various perceptual determinants.

Under conventional Rorschach interpretations each of the masters exhibited responses which would be scored as pathological. These parallel patterns involved: (1) an "unusually high shading responsivity" -- such as "diffuse cloudiness" -- suggesting that one is "at the mercy of the environment;" (2) "amorphous form responsivity" -- which fails to perceive in a way that objectifies the field into definite objects and patterns -- suggesting that one has lost a sense of boundaries and is manifesting signs of depression and anxiety; and (3) "(with certain exceptions) inanimate movement responsivity," suggestive of "infantile intrapsychic tension" and/or "hostile and uncontrollable impulses." In short, from a psychological, and therefore normative, point of view each of the protocols reflected a disintegrated and disintegrating personality pattern.

Jonte-Pace put the protocols into what she termed "a spiritual rather than a psychological context." In a spiritual context the responses of shading, amorphous form, and inanimate movement take on different meaning. She identifies these determinants as mystical, namely: "reality is in constant flux; self-environment boundaries are blurred; and the experience of nothingness or groundlessness is common." In spiritual experience, ordinary perception is deautomatized and then resymbolized primarily in terms which the particular culture has used to interpret and explain the cosmos.

While the data she reports are limited, the implications are suggestive. I link that deautomatized pattern of the spiritual masters to what is now being identified in explorations of the microstructure of cognition as subsymbolic parallel, distributed processing (Rumelhart et al [1986] 1987). In effect, our older brain constitutes our common heritage, that which we share with every person regardless of culture, class, race, or gender. That older brain also connects us with other mammals, with other organisms, with every part of the physical universe.

Our newer brain constitutes our particular heritage, that which we share with some other mammals and which distinguishes us from all other organisms. Instincts and intuitions call forth consciousness and call for articulation. We cannot **not** interpret what we observe. The nonconscious mind attends to maintaining an inner equilibrium and our conscious mind attends to developing an outer rationale. We give voice to what we experience.

Most people tend to rely upon or prefer various parts of the whole more than utilizing the whole itself. That has led to the popular characterization of "right brained people in a left brained world" or "left brained people in a right brained world," depending upon the particular values a person espouses. Whether we use brain processes or belief patterns to understand and interpret our experience, we need all our brains and the God of us all.

Putting the Pieces Together

In 1952, Paul MacLean proposed that the frontal lobes of the two hemispheres are "the seat of the highest human faculties, such as foresight and concern for the consequences and meaning of events." But he went on to suggest that the new brain -- with its two hemispheres -- may have these functions of conscious intentionality and assessment "by virtue of intimate connections between the frontal lobes and the limbic system" (quoted by Konner [1982] 1983, 147).

The years since are proving MacLean correct. The limbic level does have extensive and intricate projections into the neocortex (MacLean 1985). Emotional meaning and propositional explanation combine. The head directs our destiny even as it is out of the heart that our destiny is decided. The neocortex acts in accordance with what the older cortex determines to be necessary for the long term survival of humanity.

Figure 9 shows the connections between the brain and belief. I think of this as an expanding circle of complexity. At each level we find an integration of complementary processes, from the inner core representing the limbic system to the outer circle suggestive of the cosmos itself:

(1) in the limbic system is the integrated action of arousal in the amygdala and relaxation in the septum;[1]

(2) conscious life extends outward by means of left brain item-by-item and step-by-step processes and right brain processes of all-at-once and leaps of imagination;

(3) in the next circle are found the cognitive representations in left mind vigilant-rationality and right mind responsive-relationality;

(4) these mental process move outward into patterns of belief which name and demand (analyze) in proclamation and which embrace (immerse) and envision in manifestation; and finally,

(5) in the emerging, evolving, rippling of what matters most in this human cosmos we find the world-integrating mysticism of limbic input and the world-fullfilling action of the new brain. The Godlike brain calls us forth as creatures "made in the image and likeness of God" and entrusts us with the care of the created order of which we a part (Genesis 1:26-27).

That rippling effect of differentiated reciprocity implies these features are parallel at each level of analysis. From the autonomic nervous system to cultural systems of belief I have placed arrows moving back and forth from arousal-to-amygdala-to-items-to-vigilant-to-names and from relaxation-to-septum-to leaps-to-rela-

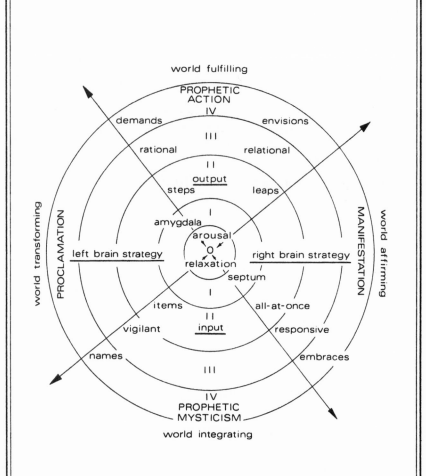

FIGURE 9. Circle Continuum of Complexity of Consciousness.

tional-to-envisions as a way of suggesting our destiny is grounded in our origin. The whole brain is needed for full human activity.

That rippling outward into the human cosmos paradoxically reaches into evolutionary adaptation. The transcendent emerges in two ways: (1) upward in ever more complex levels of organization of the new brain, and (2) downward in the subcortical integration of the old brain. In the language of the mystical tradition, the inward is outward and the outward is inward. For in God, there is neither outer nor inner. There is only God and all that is therein.

Early Renaissance theologian Nicholas of Cusa (1401?-1464) insisted that God is to be known only "beyond the coincidence of contradictories . . . and nowhere this side thereof" (Cusa 1928, 44). God is not one of the poles of any pair of opposites (Robinson 1967, 139-140) -- not amygdalar tension or septal relaxation, not left mind logic or right mind intuition, not proclamation or manifestation, not outer or inner, not matter or meaning. As Augustine put the issue of the whole being more than the parts themselves: "Neither art thou [Oh God] the mind itself. For thou art the Lord God of the mind" (Augustine 1955, Bk. X, XXV, 223).

I use the brain as both a metaphor for God and an analogy of God. As a metaphor, the brain is not God. Despite their dissimilarity, they inform each other. As an analogy, the brain connects us to God. Despite the similarity in their structure and function, the two "realities" are distinguishable. In thinking of the brain as an analogical metaphor for God, God is not reduced to left brain rationality. That would lead only to an atheistic denial of mystery. Nor is God contained in a right brain relationality. That would result only in a pantheistic engulfing by mystery. The reciprocity nature of the brain -- at every level of organization -- suggests a reciprocity nature in God.

This idea of reciprocity within the brain and within God is close to the "dialectical theism" expounded by theologian John Macquarrie. It is quite unlike the static rationality of "classical" theology.

Macquarrie's special "logic of the infinite" discloses a "dialectic of opposites" (Macquarrie [1984] 1987), after the pattern of Nicholas. As Cusa stated: "God embraces everything, even contradictions" (quoted by Macquarrie [1984] 1987, 99). Thus God is characterized with a mosaic of contradictions -- being and nothing, the one and the many, knowable and incomprehensible, transcendent and immanent, unaffected and affected by the world, eternal and temporal. But the idea of God is "an interpretative concept, meant to give us a way of understanding the relating to reality as a whole" (Marquarrie [1984] 1987, 29). In that respect the dialectic between contradictions is an organic view of reality. Everything is affected by everything and affects everything (Macquarrie [1984] 1987, 109).

The dialectical pattern between one feature and another appears similar to the reciprocal integration of brain processes. The whole is a unity and the parts reveal an internal relatedness. In the brain we can distinguish between rapid beta waves and slow alpha waves, yet these are held together and integrated by the brain as a functioning whole. Just as the concept brain gives us a way of understanding and relating to the whole of what we know, so the concept God serves a similar interpretive focus. Each idea provides coherence and accords with experience.

In the metaphor of the Nasrudin story about which is more important the sun or the moon, neither is more important. Moon and sun are parts of the solar system. In fact, no moon, no solar system; no sun, no solar system. Neither amygdala nor septum is more important. Nor is a vigilant logic less important than a responsive intuition. Every part plays a part and every part is necessary to the whole and for the whole.

Consciousness comes with the development of the neocortex. However, we must "intend" -- or choose -- to be what we are. At the level of our embeddedness in nature our nonconscious minds -- reptilian and mammalian -- make us be what we are in the long evolutionary scheme of things. At the level of our emergence into culture our conscious mind -- neocortex -- demands that we become what we are in the midst of the history which is ours. We make sense of our sensibilities by the making of meaning. Interpretations must fit with intuition and instinct. And that fit requires that we fulfill our cultural inheritances by integrating these with our genetic inheritance.

Under normal circumstances each mind acts with the whole brain involved. No matter which strategy we choose, or which hemisphere takes the lead over the other, full consciousness is present. Sometimes we rely only on one strategy or even one representational system, such as hearing or seeing. At other times we use the alternate strategy and additional representational systems, such as sensing and smelling. Except under conditions of impairment or stress, we draw upon input from all parts of the brain.

Language reflects a translation of subsymbolic (parallel distributed) processing into symbolic (sequential abstract) codes of communication. These re-presentations from sensory perception into symbolic expression constitute maps of reality. They are not reality itself (Bandler and Grinder 1975; Grinder and Bandler 1976). In the transformation of subsidiary awareness into images and on into symbols and concepts, the brain reduces a vast amount of information to simplier data. It organizes what it knows into manageable form. The conscious mind lives according to its map instead of the territory.

In the desert experience -- withdrawal from society -- or in the experience of being a stranger, our maps no longer help. We have given up or lost the bearings which come with our being creatures of habit. We cannot depend upon the habits in which we are so practiced. Under these conditions the left brain is useless and the right brain takes the lead.

In desert-like experiences if we have chosen to de-structure our everyday life, then the withdrawal becomes an experience of freshness -- freedom from the constraints of ordinary left brain time and space.

In stress if we are thrust into an uncertain context, then the loss of orientation turns into a nightmare of anxiety -- an overload of input which can result in a runaway limbic system unable to maintain its equilibrium.

Situations of excitement or anxiety often evoke an encounter with God. In terms of brain process, coming upon or finding God involves that other part of ourselves which is waiting or wanting to be found so as to become a part of something more than itself. That other part most likely means participation in the life of the whole -- a septal relaxation of survival reactions. For individuals who have identified themselves too closely with others, that other part waiting or wanting to be found requires a differentiating of themselves from others -- an amygdalar arousal of self awareness. In either instance -- courage to be as a part of the whole or courage to be as oneself -- we become freer than we were under the ordinary consciousness of our map of the way things are.

The whole brain engages all levels of brain organization, draws upon all sensory systems, and balances tension and relaxation in the service of optimal adaptation. In the metaphor of Pentecost, people hear and see and feel (Acts 2:1-4). As the spiritual masters modelled, their major sensory systems processed information with fresh perception. In the metaphor of the heavenly Jerusalem, every mind can lead us into the whole of reality (Revelation 21:12, 21, 25-26). There are twelve gates into New Reality, and in the injunction of Jesus, we are to love "with all our mind." Godlike brains in a Godlike world!

Assessing Conscious Reality

That perspective of Godlike brains enables us to view consciousness on a continuum. We range between a crippled and constricted use of the brain to a creative and expanded use. While we tend to exhibit a dominant pattern of brain activity, we also give evidence of significant and fluctuating variation (Ashbrook 1984c, 85-91).

At the regressive end of the continum of consciousness our minds are deficient or disturbed. Under these conditions we use only one part of the circle of consciousness. Just as drowsiness or drunkenness or anxiety makes it difficult to sustain attention, so our use of one strategy or one sensory system leaves us with inadequate or conflicting information.

At the creative end of the continuum of consciousness our minds -- like the spiritual masters -- combine subsymbolic and symbolic processing in a differentiated, integrated, and synergistic way. Ordinary life is transformed. Here we find paradigm shifts, for instance when Martin Luther insisted that Scripture was more important than tradition or when the theory of quantum physics went beyond Newtonian physics.

Between regression and creativity we function in a more ordinary everyday way. Here the various processes of brain and belief supplement each other, depending upon the nature of the task. Adequate functioning requires the whole brain.

Yet the evidence suggests a reciprocity of components and a division of labor. Under normal conditions, one hemisphere takes the lead over the other. It responds milliseconds faster, depending upon perception of the nature of the task (Levy and Trevarthen 1976). Further, when one half is activated, the other is suspended (Galin and Ornstein 1972; Galin [1976] 1977, 42-45). In activity triggered by a rational strategy, the left brain shows active beta and the right quiet alpha. Conversely, in activity triggered by a relational strategy, the right brain shows active beta and the left quiet alpha. When one side is "on," the other side is "off."

In split brain operations the cutting of the corpus callosum showed what happens when the two halves do not communicate. The fewer the connections, the greater the confusion. The operation put people "more at the mercy of uncontrollable surges of hemispheric preponderance and to that extent [they are] handicapped in [their] ability to select strategies to fit a given situation." Patients were left with "an extreme and rigid right or left hemispheric approach" (Kinsbourne and Smith 1974, 288-289).

Neuroscientist Michael Gazzaniga described pitching horseshoes with a split brain patient (Gazzaniga 1970, 107). In the midst of their match, the patient's right hemisphere -- the emotional reactive half -- suffered an electrical explosion. It reacted with violence. With his left hand he grabbed an axe lying on the ground and started after Gazzaniga.

Gazzaniga ran, realizing that was not the moment to explain the complexity of brain function. The patient, however, grabbed his own left wrist with his right hand. His left hemisphere, unaffected by the seizure, acted to restrain the other side. A battle ensued -- right hand restraint versus left hand fury.

The account dramatizes conflicting input. We all experience moments of confusion. Each hemisphere processes different information. Like St. Paul, we do not understand our own actions for we experience ourselves wanting to act one way and find ourselves acting the opposite (Romans 7:15-17). What the operation accomplished structurally in disconnecting the two halves, anxiety and stress accomplish functionally. Information from the two hemispheres becomes fragmented and conflicting, inadequate and misleading.

I think of such conflict as a lack of synchronization between the survival mechanism of the amygdala and the sharing mechanism of the septum. The imbalance results in a desperate attempt by the interpreting left brain to make sense of information which is discordant at the subcortical level. Thinking is impaired; memory is disturbed; attention is too narrow or too broad; the immune system is disrupted (Selye 1976; Rossi 1986, 57-67; Gazzaniga 1988, 196-210; Ornstein and Sobel, 1987).

This is especially poignant for people who have been abused as children -- sexually, physically, emotionally -- or suffer severe stress resulting in post traumatic syndromes. Symptoms include: (1) psychic numbing, (2) intrusive recollections of the traumatic events, and (3) a hypervigilance and lateralization of left hemisphere activity (Brende 1982). Recovery requires the establishment of a stable and trusting relationship which gradually allows a more integrated balancing of threatening and relaxing input (Brende and McCann, 1984).

At the conscious level, information says everything is "all right" -- which activates sepatal relaxation -- and at the emotional level information says everything is "all wrong" -- which activates amygdalar arousal. The confusion makes for psychic uncertainty and biological disturbance. A person cannot trust one's own experience. One oscillates between approaching the situation and avoiding it. The limbic system's consolidating attention, emotion, learning, and memory are in a runaway condition, unable succesfully to mediate between the outer world and the inner world.

The hippocampus transfers information from short-term memory into long-term memory (Gazzaniga 1988, 204). We can chart the course of such transfer by attending to our pattern of sleeping and dreaming (Winson [1985] 1986). Rapid eye movement sleep (REM) is the condition which occurs about every 90 to 120 minutes, three or four times a night. In this condition of suspended animation we experience our most vivid and bizarre dreams. Under our eye lids our eyes move as though we are watching a movie. Because this imaging process appears central to memory, survival, and transforming new experience into familiar experience, infants have the largest ratio of REM sleep and elderly people the lowest ratio. Every significant change in a person's routine will activate REM sleep.

I infer from this evidence that creative consciousness requires: (1) an encounter with novel events, and (2) the incorporative process of REM sleep. We combine something unfamiliar with what is old to create an unexpected-though-recognizable reality. The process of assimilating emotionally powerful new experience seems to take about three years (Winson [1985] 1986), even under the best of circumstances. That is why people find it takes three to four years to assimilate major changes in their lives -- be they death, divorce, moves, or successes. The increase in REM sleep -- reflecting novel input -- and the appearance of nightmares -- reflecting disturbed input -- are understandable mechanisms.

Genuine integration, it seems, is more subcortical than cortical. The pattern making right brain and the interpretive left brain collaborate in putting together information which is visceral and visual -- what Polanyi (1966) referred to as "the tacit dimension" of subsidiary awareness. But the consolidated memory comes only with a balance in the limbic system. We cannot "will" the integration; we can only "attend" to the process of information assimilation. Integration comes in the old brain, not the new brain.

We are conscious of discrepant information whenever we cannot "make sense" of situations. Logical explanations do not help. Choices are inadequate as well as inconceivable. Under these circumstances most of us give up, only to discover after a night's sleep or a time out, a solution comes to us. Under extreme stress people sometimes "hear" a voice or "see" a vision which resolves the dilemma. Since life is on the side of life, such resolutions are adaptive. If we can relax, our subsymbolic image processing produces a resolution -- what can be viewed as a higher order synthesis.

The key to full consciousness is the whole circle of consciousness, from the subsymbolic system to the symbolic system of the culture. The rippling consequences are always emergent and never stereotyped. We possess Godlike brains because we live in a Godlike reality.

Some interpreters of full consciousness argue for a "multimind" (Ornstein 1986), "the social brain" (Gazzaniga 1985), or a "society of mind" made up of ever-smaller agents which themselves are mindless (Minsky [1985] 1986). I agree with these views of variability in the brain. They help substantiate the viability of many "frames of mind," to use the language of cognitive psychology (Gardner 1983), or encourage Christian tolerance, to use the language of Pauline theology (Jewett 1982). With a full flow of information the cooperative, balancing strategies of left and right minds and new mind/old brain "combine to program a unitary pattern of behavior" (Kinsbourne 1982). People use whatever works best in the situation they find themselves. Every response draws upon the whole brain.

From a theological point of view, the uttered word of proclamation requires the renewing power of presence if that explanatory vigilance is not to become merely "abstract and cerebral" (Ricoeur 1978). For those of us in the Christian tradition, only the incarnation, as Ricouer put it, "ceaselessly reinterpreted gives this word something to say." That "something" is addressed to "our imagination and our heart" as well as to "our understanding and will . . . in short, to the whole human being" (Ricoeur 1978, 35).

In prophetic mysticism and prophetic action, saving the world by transforming the world is integrated into evolutionary adaptive behavior. In parallel fashion, savoring the world by affirming the world is fulfilled in our being part of the whole family of humanity. Caring for the world, thereby, expresses both saving and savoring in concrete historical situations.

Summary

The path from split brains to basic beliefs is both simple and complex. It is simple in that there is a continuity, a pattern of parallel processing from lower to higher levels of life. (Table 7) These all function on behalf of persons-in-community. There is no one way to be whole minded. For that we need humanity itself -- many minds, many hearts; living in one universe, on one earth, as one family. The issue of the brain is never an individual matter. No brain is Godlike in itself.

TABLE 7 ORGANIZATION, BRAIN, MIND AND BELIEF

Level of Analysis, discourse domain, & universe of influence	Strategy	
	Left Brain Active Process	Right Brain Receptive Process

0 autonomic
  nervous system
	arousal
	(ergotropic)
	sympathetic
	  system
		relaxation
		(trophotropic)
		parasympathetic
		  system

I limbic system	amygdala	septum
II hemisphere process	item-by-item step-by-step	all-at-once leaps of imagination
III mind activity	vigilant-rational	responsive-relational

IV belief pattern	proclaims by
	  naming &
	  analyzing
		manifests by
		  embracing &
		  envisioning

	prophetic mysticism (within the self)	
	prophetic action (in society)	
V synergistic	world trans- forming	world affirming
	world-integrating	
	world-fulfilling	

Whole brain belief originates in the old brain's evolutionary adaptation to our genetic inheritance and in the new brain's conscious intention to fulfill the will of God through our cultural inheritance. That mystical connection with the physical universe directs our action in the immediate contexts in which we live and move and have our being. We identify the oppressive forces in culture -- a left brain transforming of the world by naming and analyzing the truth of what is. We simultaneously engage the liberating power in the world -- a right brain affirming of the world by immersion in a concrete context and imagining "a new heaven and a new earth."

From a theological perspective no one is "created in the image and likeness of God," complete in oneself. According to Genesis 1:26-28, generic humanity is plural -- "them" -- "male and female" (Bird 1981; 1988). No one carries the whole image of God. We need each other. By ourselves we are only a half begotten image of God.

From a neuroscience perspective there is no such thing as "the brain." There are only individual "brains." Each brain bears its own marks of meaning, its own evolved network of synaptic transactions which make for unique perceptual realities. Every cognitive category is the imaginative construction of visceral and visual perceptions. Cultural expressions consist of prototypical exemplars of shared meaning, not propositional and substantial entities of eternal truth. By ourselves we are only one brain among many brains.

My point is simple: each of us has a brain unique to her or himself. Yet each brain links us to the universe. Not "the brain" but "brains."

This is as obvious and oblique as in the story of Nasrudin smuggling donkeys from Persia to Greece. Not "the image of God" in individuals but only in humanity, only in male-and-female, only in *homo sapiens*.

This is as systemic and intricate as the story of Nasrudin supposedly arguing that the moon is more important than the sun because "at night we need the light more." Not physical or mental, not body or mind, not brain or belief but only every part in an indivisible reality of making the whole meaning-ful.

We ignore the brain's uniqueness to our peril.

We believe God's graciousness for the possibility of our becoming the genuinely human beings that we are born to be.

Neuroscientist Candice Pert pioneered in identifying opiate receptors which mediate altered states of consciousness and the brain's natural pain relievers (Hooper and Teresi 1986 1987, 76-80, 83-85, 88-92, 101-102). Molecules and mystical states are one reality -- the biological brain and the cognitive mind, the old brain and the new mind, neither higher nor lower, better nor worse, more important nor less important. When asked whether she felt any sense of awe about the universe as Einstein had expressed when contemplating the laws of the universe, she said:

> No, I don't feel an awe for the brain. I feel an awe for God. I see in the brain all the beauty of the universe and its order -- constant signs of God's presence. I'm learning that the brain obeys all the physical laws of the universe. It's not anything special. And yet it's the most special thing in the universe (Hooper and Teresi 1986, 1987, 390).

The beginning of "the brain and belief" is ever an act of faith, a sense of awe for God. So the fulfillment of "the brain and belief" is ever an expression of sensibility, an orderliness which is "not anything special" and yet is "the most special thing in the universe."

After my sabbatical lecture on "Can The Brain Speak of God?" and an evening's discussion with faculty colleagues, Professor Larry G. Murphy sent me a copy of a traditional pygmy hymn which reminded him of the event. I close with it because it sings the hymn that I would sing:

> In the beginning was God,
> Today is God,
> Tomorrow will be God.
> Who can make an image of God?
> He has no body.
> He is as a word which comes out of your mouth.
> That word! It is no more,
> It is past, and still it lives!
> So is God.

NOTES

1. I have not dealt with the biological framework in terms of the neurotransmitter systems which subserve each sphere of consciousness and the coordinating system which holds the hemispheres in a common process. Three of these systems appear to be particularly distinctive in that regard: (a) norepinephrine in relation to the nondominant (right) hemisphere, (b) dopamine in relation to the dominant (left) hemisphere, and (c) serotonin in relation to interhemispheric (corpus callosum collaboration) activity. For an extended description and analysis see Harris (1986). A more easily understood analysis of cognitive and biochemical communication can be found in Rossi (1986) and in Ornstein and Sobel (1987). In developing the new language of mind-body communication Rossi explains the autonomic nervous system, the endocrine system, the immune system, and the neuropetide system and how we can access each and the influence of each on our health and wellbeing.

A GLOSSARY for BELIEF

ANALOGICAL: a way of referring to God by way of concepts and inferences drawn from the natural, finite, created world.

ATTRIBUTES OF GOD: characteristic ways of referring to and defining the nature of God.

CATHOLIC: refers to what is universal, orthodox, true, and shared. Prior to the Protestant Reformation it meant the historical tradition of the Latin West, namely, Roman.

CATHOLIC SUBSTANCE: the phrase of Tillich which emphasizes the concrete expression of Spiritual Presence.

CHRISTOLOGY: the part of Christian doctrine which focuses on the meaning of God's revelation in Jesus Christ.

COSMOLOGY: the "doctrine of the world" or that inquiry which focuses on the origin and nature of the universe.

CREATION: the view that all things are ultimately dependent on the Creator God as the one transcendent reality.

DIALECTICAL: a way of reasoning based on a pattern of logical development and contrast.

DUALISM: a philosophical view which holds that matter and mind are two separate and irreducible substances.

EMPIRICAL: an inductive approach to knowledge which looks to and is derived from concrete experience and which in theology involves inferences about God drawn from "facts" in the public domain.

EMPIRICAL THEOLOGY: an effort to develop theology on the basis of human experience and scientific knowledge.

EPISTEMOLOGY: the sources, scope, and criteria of knowledge; attention to the power of human reason to grasp basic truth and the evidence of empirical data based on the senses.

ESCHATOLOGY: that part of Christian doctrine which deals with the final end and purpose of human life in God.

ETERNAL: that which is not subject to time and so is above time and space.

FAITH: one's basic and intentional orientation to life in contrast to belief which involves conceptual assent; basically, the centrality of a whole response of unconditioned trust, most properly, only in relationship to God ultimately.

HERESY: that which the Church defined as contrary to its established beliefs.

KAIROS: a Greek word used in the New Testament to refer to nonmeasurable and meaningful time, e.g., "fulness of time" or "ripe time," in contrast to clock time.

KERYGMA: the Greek word meaning "to proclaim" the good news of the Gospel, i.e., "the preaching" of the Church.

LOGOS: the Greek word for reason, order, or mind of God, which the Church used to identify and understand God's action in Christ.

MANIFESTATION: the constellation of beliefs and practices that has preverbal disclosures of wonder, power, and mystery in and through natural and symbolic expressions as the primary focus of meaning.

METAPHORICAL: a way of thinking which focuses on the surplus meaning in language and by so doing identifies basic similarities between referents even as it recognizes dissimilarities.

NATURAL THEOLOGY: an approach to understanding God apart from special revelation and on the basis of general revelation, i.e., experience and reason.

ONTOLOGY: the inquiry into the rational, coherent, and necessary nature of the universe, i.e., the nature of ultimate Being.

ORTHODOXY: that which is taken to be correct, normative, and right in terms of belief. It also refers to those Eastern Churches related to Constantinople.

PATRISTIC: that period and those theologians ("the Fathers") of the early church between the first and 8th century.

PHENOMENOLOGY: a method of understanding which identifies the basic structure given in the phenomena of experience and brackets assumptions as to causal factors.

PROCLAMATION: the constellation of beliefs and practices that has the centrality of the spoken Word, instructions and imperatives, as the primary focus of meaning.

PROPHETIC-HISTORICAL: the constellation of beliefs and practices, according to Tracy, that has practical transformative action, that which calls into question existing institutions and ideologies as the primary focus of meaning.

PROTESTANT PRINCIPLE: the phrase of Tillich which emphasizes the protest against every claim to ultimacy made on behalf of any finite reality.

REDEMPTION: God acting to save or restore the relationship which has been broken with God because of Humanity's sin and rebellion.

SACRAMENTAL: the view of life that God is present, embodied, and communicated in and through the concrete world. A sacrament is a specific rite which mediates God's grace uniquely, an "outward and visible sign of an inward and spiritual reality."

SCHOLASTICISM: the pattern of Medieval thought that assumed a rational structure to reality and, therefore, self-evident knowledge and which devoted itself to detailed elaboration of that universal rationality based on the authority of the Latin Fathers and of Aristotle (and his commentators).

SYMBOL: an image or object that bears and creates special meaning that is concrete and tangible without being literal and limited. According to Tillich, symbols, in contrast to signs, participate in that which they express.

THEOLOGY: the attempt to discover, define, defend, and share the truth implied by the experience of the faith of the Church. More generally, it is a way of thinking about the nature and meaning of the divine that is both rational and systematic.

GLOSSARY for the BRAIN

ACTIVATION: the arousal process of the brainstem systems

ADAPTATION: any beneficial modification of the organism that is necessary to meet environmental demands.

AFFECT: emotional response.

ALPHA WAVES: the long, slow, synchronized brain waves (8-13 cycles per second) recorded by EEG during wakefulness which indicate nonattention and relaxation.

AMYGDALA: the almond-shaped structures in the limbic system thought to motivate emotions involving survival of the self, such as aggression, fight-flight, and the struggle for food.

ANTERIOR: situated further toward the front of the cerebral cortex, as opposed to posterior.

APHASIA: a class of disorders affecting the ability to translate experiences into verbal symbols rather than actually involving organs of speech.

AROUSAL: the physiological condition of behavioral alertness activating the sympathetic adrenal response of the fight-flight pattern of the autonomic nervous system.

ASSOCIATION CORTEX: those parts of the brain which are neither sensory nor motor but have the function of associating or integrating the incoming sensations with the outgoing motor functions.

ASYMMETRY: a term which refers to structural or functional differences between the left and right hemispheres.

ATTEND: the intentional selection of, and focus on, certain aspects of experience to the exclusion of other aspects.

ATTENTIONAL DOMINANCE: cognitive patterns by which information processing is handled according to the expectancy set either by the left or the right hemisphere.

AUDITORY: involves the sense of hearing.

AUTONOMIC NERVOUS SYSTEM: a part of the nervous system somewhat independent of the central nervous system and so somewhat independent of voluntary control. It includes the sympathetic and parasympathetic systems which regulate breathing, heart rate, blood pressure, unintentional movement, and hormone secretions.

BETA WAVES: the fast, short brain waves (12-18 cycles per second) reflective of mental activity and arousal.

BILATERAL: each hemisphere is the mirror image of the other structurally and functionally, which means that a function is distributed equally across both hemispheres, in contrast to being confined to one.

BRAINSTEM: the enlarged bulbous area of the upper part of the spinal cord which is responsible for carrying sensory information from the various parts of the body to the thalamus and motor information from the cortex to the centers in the stem and spinal cord. It encases the reticular activating system.

BROCA'S AREA: the area of the brain in the left frontal cortex associated with articulated or spoken speech.

CENTRAL NERVOUS SYSTEM: the brain and spinal cord which are responsive to conscious or deliberate intention.

CEREBRAL CORTEX: the outer, convoluted gray matter of the two hemispheres necessary for higher cognitive activity and constituting the top 80% of the human brain.

CEREBRAL HEMISPHERES: the two large halves of the brain which rest on top of the brainstem and are separated by a cleft (fissure) which runs lengthwise between them.

CEREBRUM: the largest part of the brain, which in humans perceives sensory input, organizes thought and memory, and controls voluntary activity. Another name for the cerebral cortex.

COGNITIVE PROCESSES: the mental activity of perceiving, conceiving, reasoning, and judging and includes the additional intellectual aspects of remembering, attitudes, motives, etc.

COMMISSURES: the neural connections between the corresponding areas in the right and left hemispheres, the largest being the corpus callosum.

COMMISSUROTOMY: an operation cutting the connections between the two hemispheres, primarily the corpus callosum and the anterior commissure.

CONVERGENT PROCESSING: the logical cognitive process which creates order and consistency. The opposite of divergent.

CORPUS CALLOSUM: the large group of nerve fibers which connects the two halves of the brain, sending information back and forth and coordinating their activities.

CORRELATES: at the level of the brain, biological events that change as behavior changes; at the level of the mind, cognitive processes that accompany socio-psychological-cultural activities.

CORTEX: cerebral cortex

DIVERGENT PROCESSING: the fluid cognitive process which generates variety and newness. The opposite of convergent.

ELECTROENCEPHALOGRAM (EEG): a recording of electrical changes in large groups of nerves by means of attaching electrodes to the surface of the scalp.

EPILEPSY: a disturbance of the nervous system in which a damaged area in the brain produces electrical discharges (like a thunderstorm) which can result in seizures or convulsions by spreading through the brain.

FIELD DEPENDENCE: difficulty in separating a stimulus from its surrounding context. The right hemisphere is visually more field dependent than the left.

FOREBRAIN: the two cerebral hemispheres, characteristic of mammalian brains.

FRONTAL LOBES: the front part of the cerebral cortex where initiating, planning, executing, and evaluating behavior originates.

HABITUATION: the process by which a repeated stimulus loses the ability to elicit a reaction.

HEMISPHERE: a lateral half of the cerebral cortex.

HIPPOCAMPUS: the large, curved structures in the limbic system which resemble a small marine seahorse and are thought to contribute to memory.

HOLISTIC: the simultaneous processing of information in terms of a pattern or configuration of information which is more than the sum of separate pieces.

HYPOTHALAMUS: a small structure near the base of the brain which serves as the master gland mediating mind-body communication by regulating hormonal activity, hunger, thirst, temperature, sleep, sex, and autonomic nervous system integration.

LATERAL EYE MOVEMENT: a shifting of the eyes (either left or right) when responding to a task requiring selective activation of one hemisphere over the other.

LESION: brain tissue damage due to injury, disease, or surgical procedure.

LIMBIC SYSTEM: a group of functionally related subcortical structures of the brain at the border ("limbus") of the stem and the hemispheres associated with emotional and motivational behavior such as hunger, thirst, sex, fight-flight, preservation of the self (the amygdala) and continuity of the species (septum).

MOTOR AREAS: the middle areas of the cerebral cortex directly associated with motor movements.

NEOCORTEX: the outer layer of the cerebrum which is the uniquely human or rational brain capable of symbolization, intellect, and imagination.

NEURON: the basic elements of cortical tissue, i.e., the complete nerve cell which comprises the basic structural and functional elements of cortical tissue.

NEUROSCIENCE: the multidisciplinary study of the structure, chemistry, and the biological and psychological functions of the nervous system.

OCCIPITAL LOBES: the back part of the cerebral cortex that processes visual information.

OLFACTORY LOBES: the sensory parts of the brain which mediate smell and are an extension of the cerebrum.

PARASYMPATHETIC: one of the two subdivisions of the autonomic nervous system and associated with rest, relaxation and renewal.

PARIETAL LOBES: the top middle part of the cerebral cortex that processes general sensory input from the body itself.

PERIPHERAL NERVOUS SYSTEM: the parts of the nervous system apart from the central nervous system of brain and spinal cord and in contact with the environment.

POSTERIOR: situated toward the back of the cerebral cortex, as opposed to anterior or "toward the face."

PROPOSITIONAL: the capacity of language to create words and combinations of words in an infinite number of sensible statements or "propositions."

REPTILIAN BRAIN: the oldest part of the forebrain which rests on top of the brainstem and involves instinctual behavior.

RETICULAR ACTIVATING SYSTEM (RAS): the system in the brain stem which sends impulses to the thalamus and cortex, resulting in wakefulness and attention as well as giving a constant input of stimulation to maintain the resting potential just below the critical threshold of consciousness.

SENSORY AREAS: the regions in the middle of the cerebrum directly involved in receiving sensory information.

SEPTUM: the hedge-like structures in the limbic system thought to motivate behaviors related to the preservation of the species such as grooming, sociability, and cooperation.

SET: a cognitive orientation or "mind-set" of how to organize and deal with cognitive problems, a predisposition to utilize a certain strategy.

SOMATIC: relating to the body or visceral factors.

SPATIAL: orientation to visualizing or manipulating objects in space, e.g., doing a jigsaw puzzle or drawing from a perspective.

SPECIALIZATION: the location of specific cognitive functions in either the left or the right hemisphere.

SPLIT BRAIN OPERATION: the severing of the nerve fibers which carry information between the two halves of the brain.

SPLENIUM: the large posterior area of the corpus callosum across which visual and auditory information from each hemisphere is communicated to the other.

SUBCORTICAL: areas of the brain below the cerebral cortex, including the limbic system and the brain stem.

SYMPATHETIC: one of the two subdivisions of the autonomic nervous system which is activated during arousal, tension, and stress for purposes of action.

SYNERGY: the enhancement of factors so that the combination goes beyond what can be expected from the mere addition of parts.

TACHISTOSCOPE: an instrument to present visual material for fractions of a second. A subject looks at a dot in the center of the visual field and the device permits presenting images to only one hemisphere.

TEMPORAL LOBES: the parts of the lower level of the cerebral cortex which process sounds.

THALAMOCINGULATE: a division of the limbic system thought to motivate behavior related to the maintenance of familial patterns such as maternal nursing, communication contact with offspring, and play.

UNILATERAL: relevant or relating to only one side of the cerebral cortex.

UNCOMMITTED CORTEX: the newly evolved areas of the cerebral cortex which are not specifically predetermined or "committed" to sensory or motor functions.

WERNICKE'S AREA: the region next to the temporal lobe which receives and analyzes auditory information in terms of meaningful comprehension.

FURTHER STUDY

The range of literature in neuropsychology is massive, as is the case with theology. The number of references cited suggest something of the plausibility of my conviction that the brain offers clues to the nature of the universe, ourselves, and God. Hopefully, you find some references which awaken your interest in further study.

For a more organized approach, I suggest the following books. They summarize, synthesize, critique, and provide perspective on what is being considered in the areas noted. In suggesting them, I agree with Jerome Bruner that any subject can be taught with integrity at any level. Therefore, a popular book can convey basic information and insight as well as a more technical work, and in some instances better. I have selected three books in each area: a somewhat popular book, an advanced work, and a more technical volume. Choose among them according to your background and interest.

The Brain

The 3-Pound Universe: The Brain (New York: Laurel, Dell Publishing, [1986] 1987), by Judith Hooper and Dick Teresi, is the most comprehensive report of current work in the neurosciences accessible to a lay reader. The authors are seasoned science reporters. They talked with scientists in every part of the world after doing their homework of reading the literature in depth. The result is a highly personalized report of the research being conducted and the researchers doing the research.

Left Brain, Right Brain. Rev. ed. (New York: W.H. Freeman and Company, [1981] 1985), by Sally P. Springer and Georg Deutsch, is an informed and critical review of the evidence related to the two hemispheres, what in technical language is known as cerebral asymmetry. The revised edition is one-third larger than the earlier work, reflecting both the mushrooming evidence related to the topic and the continuing importance of the area. Particular attention to issues of handedness and gender, as well as some recognition of the speculative generalizations related to culture, make this of interest to the curious lay person.

Fundamentals of Human Neuropsychology. Second edition (New York: W.H. Freeman and Company, [1980] 1985), by Bryan Kolb and Ian Q. Whishaw, is used as a standard text in both undergraduate and graduate courses in physiological and cognitive psychology. While thorough in its coverage of topics, it is very readable because of the effort to simplify many of the complex issues. In the revision, more attention is given to the biological content and evolutionary principles as well as to increased clinical content and application. The information in most chapters has been updated. Much of the material can be understood at various levels of sophistication in the neurosciences.

Consciousness

The Psychology of Consciousness. Completely revised and updated edition (New York: Penguin Books, [1972, 1977] 1986), by Robert E. Ornstein, who pioneered in opening up implications of split-brain research for the lay public. The 1977 edition (New York: Harcourt Brace Jovanovich) has the most inviting format of the three. The latest edition, however, revised on the basis of feedback from thousands of readers of the earlier volumes, combines an updated text, the original and fascinating Sufi stories of the incomparable Nasrudin, with basic articles which had appeared in Ornstein's edited volume on *The Nature of Human Consciousness: A Book of Readings* (San Francisco: W.H. Freeman and Company, 1973). It is unmatched in combining the excitement being generated by a new consciousness of consciousness and the empirical data upon which those implications are being developed.

The Universe Within: A New Science Explores The Human Mind (New York: A Touchstone Book Published by Simon and Schuster, [1982] 1983), by Morton Hunt, a long time science writer specializing in psychology. In a technical yet readable way he presents a thorough, informative, and imaginative review of how human intellectual ability, or mind, makes us radically different from other forms of life. The complexity of the cognitive sciences becomes accessible.

The Mind's New Science: A History of the Cognitive Revolution (New York: Basic Books, Inc., 1985), by research psychologist Howard Gardner, provides a full-scale history, critique, and a suggested direction for an integrated cognitive science. He develops these prospects as a result of the last twenty years of an interdisciplinary quest for mind, the nature of knowledge, and how it is represented in the mind.

Body-Mind Healing

Minding the Body, Mending the Mind (Reading, MA: Addison-Wesley Publishing Company, Inc., 1987), by Joan Borysenko, with Larry Rothstein and Forward by Herbert Benson, integrates her own personal, spiritual understanding with her work as co-founder and director of the Mind/Body Clinic at New England Deaconness Hospital, thereby forging a new medical synthesis known as psychoneuroimmunology. Hers is a warm, practical, carefully documented work on a program in which one learns the relaxation response, reframes life's problems to let go of anger and guilt, and to open oneself to love and peace.

The Healing Brain: Breakthrough Discoveries About How the Brain Keeps Us Healthy (New York: A Touchstone Book, 1987), by Robert Ornstein and David Sobel, reports on the rapidly accumulating evidence of how the brain maintains stability -- within the body and by simplifying external stimuli -- for the sake of managing health.

The Psychobiology of Mind-Body Healing: New Concepts of *Therapeutic Hypnosis* (New York: W.W. Norton & Company, Inc., 1986), by Ernest Lawrence Rossi, identifies a "mind-gene connection" in which thoughts and emotions can facilitate healing. In addition to marshalling much of current research in the psychobiology of the autonomic, endocrine, immune, and neuropeptide systems, he specifies procedures enabling a person to convert symptoms into signals of significance in and for healing.

Theology

Models of God: Theology for an Ecological, Nuclear Age (Philadelphia: Fortress Press, 1987), by Sallie McFague, goes beyond her argument in *metaphorical theology* (1982) for "the importance in religion of imagistic language as the base and funding for conceptual, theological language," (which I associate with right hemisphere language and the language of change) to a "*remythologizing* of the relationship between God and the world" in such metaphorical models as "God as mother, lover, and friend of the world."

Sexism And God-Talk: Toward A Feminist Theology (Boston: Beacon, 1983), by Rosemary Radford Ruether, criticizes the patriarchal elitism which has excluded or subordinated women's participation in religious experience. She challenges the reader to a fuller vision of humanity in a positive, egalitarian religion in which relational values, indicative of right brain activity, are integrated with rational values, indicative of left brain values.

The Analogical Imagination: Christian Theology and The Culture of Pluralism (Chicago: The University of Chicago Press, [1981] 1986), by David Tracy, spells out in detail the family resemblances, or belief trajectories, of proclamation, manifestation, and prophetic action as part of his case for the use of religious classics in public discourse.

Bibliography

Abailard, Pierre. 1954. Historia Calamitatum. The Story of Abelard's Adversities. A trans. with notes by J.T. Muckle. With a preface by Etienne Gilson. Toronto: The Pontifical Institute of Medieval Studies.

Abba, R. "Name." In The Interpreter's Dictionary of The Bible: K-Q, ed. George A. Buttrick, 500-508. New York: Abingdon Press.

Alter, Robert. 1981. The Art of Biblical Narrative. New York: Basic Books.

Anchin, Jack C. and Donald J. Kiesler, eds. 1982. Handbook of Interpersonal Psychotherapy. New York: Pergamon Press.

Anderson, Bernard. 1967. Creation Versus Chaos: The Reinterpretation of Mythical Symbolism in the Bible. New York: Association Press.

Anderson, B.W. 1962a. "Creation." In The Interpreter's Dictionary of The Bible: A-D, ed. George A. Buttrick, 725-732. New York: Abingdon Press.

Anderson, B.W. 1962b. "God, Names Of." In The Interpreter's Dictionary of The Bible: E-J, ed. George A. Buttrick, 407-417. New York: Abingdon Press.

Anderson, Mary Lou. 1986. "Presence and Transformation: A Biblical Model of Ministry." In The Brain and Ministry, ed. by James B. Ashbrook (forthcoming).

Andreasen, Roberta. 1985. The Broken Brain: The Biological Revolution in Psychiatry. New York: Basic Books, Inc.

Anselm. 1970. Proslogion. In A Scholastic Miscellany: Anselm to Ockham, ed. and trans. for the Library of Christian Classics,

Volume X, by Eugene R. Fairweather (Westminster Press): New York: The Macmillan Company.

Aquinas, Thomas. 1945. Basic Writings of Saint Thomas Aquinas, Vol.I & II. Edited and Annotated, with an Introduction by Anton C. Pegis. New York: Random House.

Ardila, Alfredo and Peggy **Ostrosky-Solis,** eds. 1984. The Right Hemisphere: Neurology and Neuropsychology. New York: Gordon and Breach.

Arendt, Hannah [1971,1977] 1978. The Life of the Mind, Vol.One Thinking. New York: Harcourt Brace Jovanovich.

Arndt, William and F. Wilbur **Gingrich.** Second edition revised and augmented by F. Wilbur Gingrich and Frederick W. Danker from Walter Bauer's Fifth Edition [1958; 1957] 1979. A Greek-English Lexicon of The New Testament and Other Early Christian Literature. Chicago: The University of Chicago Press.

Arnheim, Rudolf. 1972. Visual Thinking. Berkeley: University of California Press.

Ashbrook, James B. 1971. be/come Community. Valley Forge, PA.: Judson Press.

Ashbrook, James B. 1973. Humanitas: Human Becoming and Being Human. Nashville: Abingdon Press.

Ashbrook, James B. 1984a. "Ambiguity in Neuropsychology: A Response to Wong." Journal of Psychology and Theology Vol.12, No.4:314-319.

Ashbrook, James B. 1984b. "Neurotheology: The Working Brain and The Work of Theology." Zygon: Journal of Religion and Science Vol.19, No.3 (September): 331-350.

Ashbrook, James B. 1984c. The Human Mind and The Mind of God: Theological Promise in Brain Research. Lanham, MD: University Press of America.

Ashbrook, James B. 1985. "Brain, Mind and God." The Christian Century March 19-26:295-298.

Ashbrook, James B. 1986. "Quality of Life In A Home For The Elderly: A Systemic Approach." The Journal of Pastoral Care, Vol. XL, No.3 (September):217-232.

Ashbrook, James B. 1987a. "Between Broken Brains and Oppressive Beliefs: Troubled Minds." Chapter for a book on a public policy for psychiatry, edited by Don Browning (in press).

Ashbrook, James B. 1987b. FROM BEING TO BRAIN: Natural Theology in an Empirical Mode." Paper presented to the Science and Theology Section of the American Academy of Religion Meeting, Boston, December.

Ashbrook, James B. and Paul W. **Walaskay.** 1977. Christianity For Pious Skeptics. Nashville: Abingdon Press.

Augustine. 1955. Confessions and Enchiridion, ed. and trans. by Albert C. Outler. Philadelphia: Westminster Press.

Augustine. [1963] 1981. The Fathers of The Church: Saint Augustine The Trinity, Vol.45. Trans. by Stephen McKenna. Washington, D.C.: Catholic University of America Press.

Bakan, David. 1966. The Duality of Human Existence. Chicago: Rand McNally & Company.

Bandler, Richard and John **Grinder.** 1975. The Structure of Magic I: A Book About Language and Therapy. Palo Alto, CA: Science and Behavior Books, Inc.

Bandler, Richard and John **Grinder.** 1979. Frogs into Princes: Neuro Linguistic Programming. Ed. by John O. Stevens. Moab, Utah: Real People Press

Barbour, Ian G. 1966. Issues in Science and Religion. Englewood Cliffs, NJ: Prentice-Hall, Inc.

Bates, E. 1976. The Emergence of Symbols. New York: Academic Press.

Bear, David M. and Paul **Fedio.** 1977. "Quantitative Analysis of Intertictal Behavior in Temporal Lobe Epilepsy." Archives of Neurology Vol.34 (August):451-467.

Belenky, Mary Field, Blythe McVicker **Clinchy,** Nancy Rule **Goldberger,** and Jill Mattuck **Tarule.** 1986. Women's Ways of Knowing: The Development of Self, Voice, and Mind. New York: Basic Books.

Benderly, Beryl Lieff. 1987. The Myth of Two Minds: What Gender Means and Doesn't Mean. New York: Doubleday.

Benson, D. Frank and Eran **Zaidel,** eds. 1985. The Dual Brain: Hemispheric Specialization in Humans. New York: The Guilford Press.

Bentmann, Von Reinhard and Heinrich **Lickes** [1970, 1978] 1979. Churches of The Middle Ages. London: Cassell.

Benson, Herbert. 1975. The Relaxation Response. New York: William Morrow and Company.

Benson, Herbert. 1979. The Mind/Body Effect. New York: Simon & Schuster.

Benson, Herbert. 1984. Beyond the Relaxation Response: How to Harness the Healing Power of Your Personal Beliefs. With William Proctor. New York: Times Books.

Bess, Philip H. 1985. "Beyond Irony: Can Religion Point the Way to Architectural Renewal." This World Oct.:96-107.

Bettleheim, Bruno. 1978. The Uses of Enchantment: The Meaning and Importance of Fairy Tales. New York: Alfred A. Knopf.

Bever, Thomas G. 1975. "Cerebral Asymmetries in Humans Are Due to The Differentiation Of Two Incompatible Processes: Holistic and Analytic." Annals New York Academy of Sciences 251-262.

Bever, Thomas G., Richard R. **Hurtig,** and Ann B. **Handel** 1976. "Analytic Processing Elicits Right Ear Superiority in Monaurally Presented Speech." Neuropsychologia 14:175-181

Biersdorf, John E. 1985. Healing of Purpose: God's Call to Discipleship. Nashville, TN: Abingdon..

Bird, Phyllis. 1981. "'Male and Female He Created Them:' Gen. 1:27b In The Context of The Priestly Account of Creation." Harvard Theological Review 74:2, 129-159.

Bird, Phyllis. 1987. "Genesis 1-3 as a Source for a Contemporary Theology of Sexuality." Frederick Neumann Symposium, Princeton Theological Seminary.

Bird, Phyllis. 1988. "Sexual Differentiation and Divine Image in the Genesis Creation Texts." In Image of God and Gender Models, ed. by Kari E. Borresen (Oslo: Solum Forlag/Atantic Heights, NJ: Humanities Press, forthcoming).

Blakeslee, Thomas R. 1980. The Right Brain: A New Understanding of the Unconscious Mind and Its Creative Powers. Garden City, NY: Anchor Press/Doubleday.

Blakney, Raymond B. ed. [1941] 1957. Meister Eckhart: A Modern Translation. New York: Harper Torchbooks.

Bloom, Floyd E., Arlyne **Lazerson,** and Laura **Hofstadter.** 1985. Brain, Mind, and Behavior: An Annenberg/CPB Project. New York. W.H. Freeman and Company.

Bony, Jean. 1961. French Cathedrals. Photographs by Martin Hurlimann; descriptive notes by Peter Meyer. New York: A Studio Book, The Viking Press.

Bony, Jean. 1983. French Gothic Architecture of the 12th & 13th Centuries. Berkeley: University of California Press.

Bordo, Susan. [1986] 1987. "The Cartesian Masculinization of Thought." In Sex and Scientific Inquiry, ed. by Sandra Harding and Jean F. O'Barr (Chicago: The University of Chicago Press), 247-264.

Borysenko, Joan. 1987. Minding the Body, Mending the Mind. With Larry Rothstein. Forward by Herbert Benson. Reading, MA: Addison-Wesley Publishing Company.

Bowman, R.A. 1962. "Geneology." in The Interpreter's Dictionary of The Bible: E-J, ed. George A. Buttrick, 362-365. New York: Abingdon Press.

Bradshaw, John L. and Norman C. **Nettleton.** 1983. Human Cerebral Asymmetry. Englewood Cliffs, NJ: Prentice-Hall, Inc.

Brende, Joel Oster. 1982. "Electrodermal Responses in Post-traumatic Syndromes: A Pilot Study of Cerebral Hemisphere Functioning in Vietnam Veterans." Journal of Nervous and Mental Disorders, Vol. 170, No.6:352-361.

Brende, J.O. and I.L. **McCann.** 1984. "Regressive Experiences in Vietnam Veterans: Their Relationship to War, Post-traumatic Symptoms and Recovery." Journal of Contemporary Psychotherapy, Vol. 14, No.1 (Spring/Summer):57-75.

Brown, Barbara. 1973. New Body, New Mind: Biofeedback: New Directions for the Mind. New York: Harper & Row.

Brown, Peter. 1971. "The Rise and Function of the Holy Man." Journal of Roman Studies 61:80-101.

Brown, Peter. 1976. "Eastern and Western Christendom in Late Antiquity: a parting of the ways." In The Orthodox Churches And The West, ed. by Derek Baker, 11-16. Published for the Ecclesiastical History Society Oxford: Basil Blackwell.

Bryden, M.P. 1982. Laterality: Functional Asymmetry in the Intact Brain. New York: Academic Press.

Bryden, M.P. and R.G. Ley. 1983. "Right-Hemispheric Involvement in the Perception and Expression of Emotion in Normal Humans." In Neuropsychology of Human Emotion, ed. by Kenneth M. Heilman and Paul Satz, 6-44. New York: The Guilford Press.

Bumbar, Paul E. 1979. "Notes on Wholeness." In Aesthetic Dimensions of Religious Education, ed. by Gloria Durka & Joanmarie Smith, 47-68. New York: Paulist Press.

Burhoe, Ralph Wendell. 1973. "The Concepts of God and Soul In A Scientific View of Human Purpose." Zygon: Journal of Religion and Science, Vol. 8, No. 5. 3-4 (September-December): 412-442.

Burhoe, Ralph Wendell. 1981. Toward A Scientific Theology. Belfast: Christian Journals Limited.

Burhoe, Ralph Wendell. 1987. Personal conversation based on notes critiquing James B. Ashbrook's "From Being to Brain: Natural Theology in an Empirical Mode."

Burrell, David. 1973. Analogy and Philosophical Language. New Haven: Yale University Press.

Burrell, David. 1979. Aquinas: God & Action. London: Routledge & Kegan Paul.

Burrell, David. 1982. "Argument in Theology: Analogy and Narrative." In New Dimensions in Philosophical Theology, ed. by Carl A. Raschke, 37-52, Journal of the American Academy of Religious Studies, Vol. XLIX, Number 1.

Buzan, Tony. 1985. Use Both Sides of Your Brain. Rev. ed. New York: E.P. Dutton & Co., Inc.

Bynum, Caroline Walker. 1986. "Introduction The Complexity of Symbols." In Gender and Religion: On the Complexity of Symbols, ed. by Caroline Walker Bynum, Stevan Harrell, and Paula Richman, 1-20. Boston: Beacon Press.

Bynum, Caroline Walker. 1987. Holy Feast and Holy Fast: The Religious Significance of Food To Medieval Women. Berkeley: University of California Press.

Bynum Caroline Walker, Stevan **Harrell,** and Paula **Richman,** eds. 1986. Gender and Religion: On the Complexity of Symbols. Boston: Beacon Press.

Calvin, John. 1962. Institutes on the Christian Religion. Vol. 1. Trans. by Henry Beveridge. Grand Rapids, MI: Eerdmans Publishing Co.

Cather, Willa. 1971. Death Comes For The Archbishop. New York: Random House.

Chall, Jeanne S. and Allan F. **Mirsky,** eds. 1978. Education and The Brain: The Seventy-seventh Yearbook of the National Society for the Study of Education. Part II. Chicago: The University of Chicago Press.

Chodorow, Nancy [1978] 1979. The Reproduction of Mothering: Psychoanalysis and the Sociology of Gender. Berkeley: University of California Press.

Chopp, Rebecca S. 1986. The Praxis of Suffering: An Interpretation of Liberation and Political Theologies. Maryknoll, NY: Orbis Books.

Clift, Jean Dalby and Wallace B. **Clift.** 1984. Symbols of Transformation in Dreams. New York: Crossroad.

Cobb, John B., Jr. 1965. A Christian Natural Theology Based On The Thought of Alfred North Whitehead. Philadelphia: Westminster Press.

Cobb, John B. Jr. 1977. "Some Whiteheadian Comments." In Mind in Nature: Essays on the Interface of Science and Philosophy. Washington, D.C.: University Press of America.

Cole, Kenneth. 1986. "Hallowed Be The Mall." Drew, December, 10-12.

Colman, Arthur D. and W. Harold **Bexton,** eds. 1975. Group Relations Reader. Sausalito, CA: GREX. A.I. Rice Institute, Washington, D.C.

Colman, Arthur and Marvin H. **Geller,** eds. 1985. Group Relations Reader 2. Washington, D.C.: A.K. Rice Institute.

Coltheart, M., E. **Hull,** and D. **Slater.** 1975. "Sex Differences in Imagery and Reading." Nature 253:438-440.

Cross, Frank Moore. 1973. Canaanite Myth and Hebrew Epic. Cambridge, MA: Harvard University Press.

Cusa, Nicholas. 1928. The Vision of God. Trans. Emma Gurney Salter, with intro. by Evelyn Underhill. New York: Dutton.

d'Aquili, Eugene. 1983. "The Myth-Ritual Complex: A Biogenetic Structural Analysis." Zygon: Journal of Religion and Science Vol.18, No.3 (September):247-269.

d'Aquili, Eugene G. 1986. "Myth, Ritual, And The Archetypal Hypothesis." Zygon: Journal of Religion and Science Vol.21, No.2 (June): 141-160.

d'Aquili, Eugene G. and Charles D. **Laughlin**, Jr. 1979. "The Neurobiology of Myth and Ritual." In The Spectrum of Ritual: A Biogenetic Structural Analysis, ed. E. G. d'Aquili and D. C. Laughlin, Jr., 152-187. New York: Columbia University Press.

Dean, William. 1986. American Religious Empiricism. Albany, NY: State University of New York Press.

DeAngelis, Tori. 1987. "Computer Theorist. [David Rumelhart] nabs MacArthur prize." APA Monitor, August 28.

Deaux, Kay and Brenda **Major**. 1987. "Putting Gender into Context: An Interactive Model of Gender-Related Behavior." Psychological Review, Vol. 94, No. 3:369-389.

Deikman, Arthur J. 1969. "Deautomatization and the Mystical Experience." In Altered States of Consciousness: A Book of Readings, ed. by Charles T. Tart, 23-43. New York: John Wiley & Sons, Inc.

Denenberg, Victor H. 1983. "Animal Studies of Laterality." In Neuropsychology of Human Emotion, ed. by Kenneth M. Heilman and Paul Satz, 65-79. New York: The Guilford Press.

Denton, R.C. 1962. "Heart." In The Interpreter's Dictionary of The Bible: E-J, ed. George A. Buttrick, 549-550. New York: Abingdon Press.

Dimond, S.J. 1972. The Double Brain. London: Churchill-Livingstone.

Douglas, Mary. [1970, 1973] 1982. Natural Symbols: Explorations in Cosmology. With a new introduction. New York: Pantheon Books.

Durka, Gloria & Joanmarie Smith, eds. 1979. Aesthetic Dimensions of Religious Education. New York: Paulist Press.

Edwards, Betty. 1979. Drawing On The Right Side Of The Brain. Los Angeles: J.P. Tracher, Inc.

Edwards, Betty. 1986. Drawing on the Artist Within: A Guide to Innovation, Invention, Imagination and Creativity. New York: Simon and Schuster.

Ehrenwald, Jan. 1986. Anatomy of Genius: Split Brains and Global Minds. New York: Human Sciences Press, Inc.

Eliade, Mircea. [1954] 1959. Cosmos and History: The Myth of The Eternal Return. New York: Harper Torchbooks & The Bollingen Library.

Eliade, Mircea. 1969. The One Quest: History and Meaning in Religion. Chicago: University of Chicago Press.

Fairweather, Eugene R. 1970. A Scholastic Miscellany: Anselm to Ockham. Ed. and trans. for the Library of Christian Classics, Volume X (The Westminster Press). New York: The Macmillian Company.

Feindel, William. 1975. In Wilder Penfield, The Mystery of The Mind: A Cortical Study of Consciousness and The Human Brain, Princeton, NJ: Princeton University Press.

Feldenkrais, Moshe. 1972. Awareness Through Movement. New York: Harper & Row.

Feldman, Edward Burke. 1972. Varieties of Visual Experience. Basic edition. New York: Harry N. Abrams.

Flax, Jane. 1983. "The Patriarchal Unconscious." In Sandra Harding and Merrill Hintikka, eds., Discovering Reality: Feminist Perspectives on Epistemology, Metaphysics, Methodology, and Philosophy of Science. London: D. Reidel Publishing Company.

Flor-Henry, Pierre. 1983. Cerebral Bases of Psychopathology. Boston: John Wright - PSE, Inc.

Fox, Matthew. 1972. On Becoming a Musical Mystical Bear: Spirituality American Style. New York: Harper.

Frankenberry, Nancy. 1987. Religion and Radical Empiricism. Albany, NY: State University of New York Press.

Fromm, Erich. 1966. You Shall Be as Gods. New York: Holt, Rinehart & Winston.

Galin, David and Robert E. **Ornstein.** 1972. "Lateral Specialization of Cognitive Mode: An EEG Study." Psychophysiology 9:412-418.

Galin, David. [1976] 1977. "The Two Modes of Consciousness and the Two Halves of the Brain." In Symposium on Consciousness, Philip R. Lee, Robert E. Ornstein, David Galin, Arthur Deikman, and Charles T. Tart, 26-53. Baltimore: Penguin Books.

Gapp, Paul. 1988. "The Rise of Generic City: As the big buildings go up, the world looks more and more the same." Chicago Tribune, Section 13, March 20:4-5.

Gardner, Howard. [1974] 1976. The Shattered Mind: The Person After Brain Damage. New York: Vintage Books.

Gardner, Howard. 1983. Frames of Mind: The Theory of Multiple Intelligences. New York: Basic Books, Inc.

Gardner, Howard. 1985. The Mind's New Science: A History of the Cognitive Revolution. New York: Basic Books, Inc.

Gardner, H.W. [1953, 1954, 1956] 1958. Poems and Prose of Gerard Manley Hopkins. Selected With An Introduction and Notes. Baltimore: Penguin Books Inc.

Gazzaniga, Michael S. 1970. The Bisected Brain. New York: Appleton-Century-Crofts.

Gazzaniga, Michael S. 1974. "Cerebral Dominance Viewed As a Decision System." In Hemisphere Function in the Human Head, ed. S.J.Dimond and J.G.Beaumont, 367-382. New York: Wiley & Sons.

Gazzaniga, Michael S. 1985. The Social Brain: Discovering The Networks of The Mind. New York: Basic Books, 1985.

Gazzaniga, Michael S. 1988. Mind Matters: How the Mind and Brain Interact to Create Our Conscious Lives. With a forward by Robert Bazell. Boston: Houghton Mifflin Company Bradford Books.

Gazzaniga, Michael S. and Joseph **LeDoux.** 1978. The Integrated Mind. New York: Plenum Publishing Company.

Gendlin, Eugene T. 1962. Experiencing and the Creation of Meaning: A Philosophical and Psychological Approach to the Subject. Glencoe, IL: The Free Press.

Gendlin, Eugene T. 1978. Focusing. New York: Everest House Publishers.

Geschwind, Norman and Albert M. **Galaburda,** eds. 1984. Cebebral Dominance: The Biological Foundations. Cambridge, MA: Harvard University Press.

Geschwind, Norman and Albert M. **Galaburda.** 1985. "Cerebral Lateralization: Biological Mechanism, Associations, and Pathology: I. A Hypothesis and a Program for Research." Archives of Neurology Vol.42 (May):428-459.

Giedion, Sigfried. 1964. The Eternal Presence: The Beginnings of Architecture. A Contribution to Constancy and Change. New York: Pantheon Books, Bollingen Series, Vol.35.

Giedion, Sigfried. 1967. Space, Time and Architecture: The Growth of a New Tradition. 5th ed., rev. Cambridge, MA: Harvard University Press.

Gilligan, Carol. [1982] 1983. In a Different Voice: Psychological Theory and Women's Development. Cambridge, MA: Harvard University Press.

Glaz, Maxine. 1987. "Gender Issues in Pastoral Theology." Paper presented to the Society of Pastoral Theology, June. Denver, CO.

Glennon, L.M. 1979. Women and Dualism: A Sociology of Knowledge. New York: Longman.

Goldberg, Michael. 1981 and 1982. Theology And Narrative: A Critical Introduction. Nashville: Abingdon.

Goleman, Daniel. 1985. "Left vs. Right: Brain Function Tied to Hormone In the Womb." The New York Times, September 24, c1, c10.

Goodenough, Ward. 1987. "Evolutionary Issues on the Interface of Genes and Cultures." A paper presented at the American Academy of Science Symposium, February. Chicago, IL.

Gordon, William J.J. 1961. Synetics: The Development of Creative Capacity. New York: Collier Macmillan Publishers.

Goy, R.W. and B.S. **McEwen,** eds. 1980. Sexual Differentiation of the Brain. Cambridge: MIT Press.

Grinder, John and Richard **Bandler.** 1976. The Structure of Magic II: A Book About Communication and Change. Palo Alto, CA: Science and Behavior Books, Inc.

Grossman, Ron. 1987. "Dialogue vs. Drugs: Psychiatry's Mood Swings Between the Lab and Couch. Chicago Tribune, May 10, Sec.5, 1-4.

Guerdan, Rene'. [1957] 1962. Byzantium: Its Triumphs and Tragedy. Trans. by D.L.B. Hartley. With a preface by Charles Diehl. New York: Capricorn Books.

Halpern, Howard M. 1963. A Parent's Guide To Child Psychotherapy. New York: A.S.Barnes and Company, Inc.

Haly, Jay. 1973. Uncommon Therapy: The Psychiatric Techniques of Milton H. Erickson, M.D. New York: W.W.Norton & Company, Inc.

Hampden-Turner, Charles. 1981. Maps of the Mind: Charts and Concepts of The Mind and Its Labyrinths. New York: Collier Books.

Hanson, Paul D. 1982. The Diversity of Scripture: A Theological Interpretation. Philadelphia: Fortress Press.

Harding, Sandra and Merrill Hintikka, eds. 1983. Discovering Reality: Feminist Perspectives on Epistemology, Metaphysics, Methodology, and Philosophy of Science. London: D.Reidel Publishing Company.

Harding, Sandra and Jean F. O'Barr, eds. 1987. Sex and Scientific Inquiry. Chicago: The University of Chicago Press.

Harrington, Anne. 1987. Medicine, Mind, And The Double Brain. Princeton, NJ: Princeton University Press.

Harris, Jay E. 1986. Clinical Neuroscience: From Neuroanatomy to Psychodynamics. New York: Human Sciences Press, Inc.

Harris, Lauren Julius. 1985. "Teaching the Right Brain: Historical Perspective on a Contemporary Educational Fad." In Hemispheric Collaboration in the Child, ed. by Catherine T. Best, 262-267. Orlando, FL: Academic Press, Inc.

Hartshorne, Charles. 1967. A Natural Theology For Our Time. LaSalle, IL: Open Court.

Harvey, Van A. 1964. A Handbook of Theological Terms. New York: Macmillan Publishing Company.

Heilman, Kenneth M. and Paul Satz. 1983. Neuropsychology of Human Emotion. New York: The Guilford Press.

Heilman, Kenneth M., Robert T. Watson, and Dawn Bowers. 1983. "Affective Disorders Associated with Hemispheric Disease." In Neuropsychology on Human Emotion, ed. by Kenneth M. Heilman and Paul Satz, 45-64. New York: The Guilford Press.

Henry, James P. 1986. "Religious Experience, Archetypes, and The Neurophysiology of Emotions." Zygon: Journal of Religion and Science Vol.21, No.1 (March): 47-74.

Hoffman, Paul. 1987. "Your Mindless Brain." Discover September: 84-87.

Holyoak, Keith. 1987. "A Connectionist View of Cognition." Science Vol. 236, 22 May: 992-996.

Hooper, Judith and Dick **Teresi.** [1986] 1987. The 3-Pound Universe: The Brain. With a Foreword by Isaac Asimov. New York: Laurel, Dell Publishing Co.

Hopson, Janet. 1984. "Marian Diamond: A Love Affair with the Brain." Psychology Today (November):62-73.

Horowitz, Mardi Jon [1978] 1986. Stress Response Syndromes. Second Edition. Northvale, NJ: Jason Aronson, Inc.

Houston, Jean. 1982. The Possible Human: A Course in Enhancing Your Physical, Mental, and Creative Abilities. Los Angeles: J.P.Tracher, Inc.

Howe, Reuel. 1953. Man's Need and God's Action. Greenwich Conn.: The Seabury Press.

Hyde, J.S. 1981. "How Large Are Cognitive Gender Differences? A Meta-analysis Using w2 and d," American Psychologist 36:892-901.

Jenni, E. 1962. "Day of Judgment." In The Interpreter's Dictionary of The Bible: A-D, ed. George A. Buttrick, 783-784. New York: Abingdon Press.

Jerison, Harry J. 1985. "On the Evolution of Mind." In <u>Brain & Mind</u>, ed. by David A. Oakley, 1-31. New York: Methuen & Co.

Jewett, Robert. 1982. <u>Christian Tolerance: Paul's Message to the Modern Church</u>. Philadelphia: Westminster Press.

John of Salisbury. 1970. <u>The Policratus</u>. In <u>A Scholastic Miscellany: Anselm to Ockham</u>, ed. and trans. for the Library of Christian Classics, Volume X, by Eugene R. Fairweather (The Westminster Press). New York: The Macmillan Company.

Johnson, Mark. 1987. <u>The Body in the Mind: The Bodily Basis of Meaning, Imagination, and Reason</u>. Chicago: The University of Chicago Press.

Jonas Hans. 1974. <u>Philosophical Essays: From Ancient Creed to Technological Man</u>. Engelwood Cliffs, NJ: Prentice-Hall.

Jonte-Pace, Diane. 1987. "The Swami and the Rorschach: Projective Tests and Spiritual Disciplines." A paper presented to the Person, Culture, and Religion Section of the American Academy of Religion annual meeting in Boston, December.

Julian of Norwick. [1966] 1976. <u>Revelations of Divine Love</u>. Trans. into Modern English and with an Introduction by Clifton Walters. Baltimore: Penguin Books, Inc.

Kahler, Heinz. 1967. <u>Hagia Sophia</u>. With a chapter on mosaics by Cyril Mango. Trans. by Ellyn Childs. New York: Praeger Publishers.

Katzenellenbogen, Adolf. [1959] 1964. <u>The Sculptural Programs of Chartres Cathedral</u>. New York: W.W. Norton & Company, Inc.

Kegan, Robert. 1982. <u>The Evolving Self</u>. Cambridge, MA: Harvard University Press.

Keller, Evelyn Fox. 1983. "Gender and Science." In <u>Discovering Reality: Feminist Perspectives on Epistemology, Metaphysics, Methodology, and Philosophy of Science</u>, ed. by Sandra Harding and Merrill Hintikka, 187-205. London: D.Reidel Publishing Company.

Keller, Evelyn Fox and Christine R. **Grontkowski.** 1983. "The Mind's Eye." In <u>Discovering Reality: Feminist Perspectives on Epistemology, Metaphysics, Methodology, and Philosophy of Science</u>, ed. by Sandra Harding and Merrill Hintikka, 207-224. London: R.Reidel Publishing Company.

Kershner, John R. 1985. "Ontogeny ˙of Hemispheric Specialization and Relationship of Developmental Patterns to Complex Reasoning Skills and Academic Achievement." In <u>Hemispheric Function and Collaboration in the Child</u>, ed. by Catherine T. Best, 327-360. Orlando, FL: Academic Press, Inc.

Kessel, Dimitri. 1964. <u>Splendors of Christendom</u>. Switzerland: Edita Lausanne.

Kimura, Doreen. 1964. "Left-Right Differences in the Perception of Melodies." <u>Quarterly Journal of Experimental Psychology</u> 16:355-358.

Kimura, Doreen. 1985. "Male Brain, Female Brain: The Hidden Difference." <u>Psychology Today</u> November:50-58.

Kinsbourne, Marcel. 1981. <u>Psychology Today</u> (May):92.

Kinsbourne, Marcel. 1982. "Hemisphere Specialization and the Growth of Human Understanding." <u>American Psychologist</u> (April):411-420.

Kinsbourne, M. and W.L. **Smith,** eds. 1974. <u>Hemisphere Disconnection and Cerebral Function</u>. Springfield, IL: Charles Thomas.

Kittel, Gerhard, ed. 1964. Theological Dictionary of The New Testament. Translator and editor Geoffrey W. Bromiley. Grand Rapids MI: Wm. B. Eerdmans Publishing Company.

Kolb, Bryan and Ian Q. **Whishaw.** [1980] 1985. Fundamentals of Human Neuropsychology. Second edition. New York: W.H.Freeman and Company.

Konner, Melvin. [1982] 1983. The Tangled Wing: Biological Constraints on the Human Spirit. New York: Harper Colophon Book.

Korzybski, A. 1933. Science and Sanity. Lakeville, Conn.: The International Non-Aristotelian Library Publishing Company, 4th Edition.

Kotulak, Robert. 1988. "Redefining Humanity. Brain research focuses an agonizing reappraisal." Chicago Tribune, "Perspective," May 15, Section 4:1,4.

Koyama, Kosuke. 1976. Water Buffalo Theology. Maryknoll, NY: Orbis Books.

Kubose, Gyomay M. 1973. Zen Koans, and original sumie illustrations by Ryozo Ogura. Chicago: Henry Regency Company.

Lakoff, George. 1987. Women, Fire, and Dangerous Things: What Categories Reveal About the Mind. Chicago: The University of Chicago Press.

Lakoff, George and Mark **Johnson.** 1980. Metaphors We Live By. Chicago: The University of Chicago Press.

Leff, Gordon. 1958. Medieval Thought: Saint Augustine to Ockham. Baltimore: Penguin Books.

Levy, Jerre. 1974. "Psychobiological Implications of Bilateral Asymmetry." In Hemisphere Function in the Human Head, ed. S.J.Dimond and J.G.Beaumont, 121-183. New York: Wiley & Sons.

Levy, Jerre. 1980a. "Cerebral Asymmetry and The Psychology of Man." In The Brain and Psychology, ed. by M.C.Wittrock, 252-321. New York: Academic Press.

Levy, Jerre. 1980b. "Varieties of Human Brain Organization and the Human Social System." Zygon: Journal of Religion and Science Vol. 15, No.14 (December):351-375.

Levy, Jerre. 1983. "Language, Cognition, and the Right Hemisphere." American Psychologist 38 (May):538-541.

Levy, Jerre. 1985a. "Right Brain, Left Brain: Fact and Fiction." Psychology Today (April):38-44.

Levy, Jerre. 1985b. "Interhemispheric Collaboration: Single-Mindedness in the Asymmetrical Brain." In Hemisphere Function and Collaboration in the Child, ed. by Catherine T. Best, 11-31. Orlando, FL: Academic Press.

Levy, Jerre, Wendy Heller, Marie T. Barich, and Leslie A. Burton. 1983. "Are Variations Among Right-Handed Individuals in Perceptual Asymmetries Caused by Characteristic Arousal Differences Between Hemispheres?" Journal of Experimental Psychology: Human Perception and Performance Vol. 9, No.3 (June):329-359.

Levy, Jerre and Colwyn Trevarthen. 1976. "Metacontrol of Hemisphere Function in Human Split-Brain Patients." Journal of Experimental Psychology: Human Perception and Performance No. 2:299-312.

Levy-Agresti, Jerre and R.W. Sperry. 1968. "Differential Perceptual Capacities in Major and Minor Hemispheres." Proceedings of the National Academy of Sciences 61:1151.

Livingston, Robert B. 1978. Sensory Processing, Perception, and Behavior. New York: Raven Press.

Luria, A.R. 1973. The Working Brain: An Introduction to Neuropsychology. Trans. by Basil Haigh. New York: Basic Books, Inc.

Maccoby, Eleanor Emmons and Carol Nagy **Jacklin.** 1974. The Psychology of Sex Differences. Stanford, CA: Stanford University Press.

MacLean, Paul D. 1952. "Some Psychiatric Implications of Physiological Studies on Frontotemporal Portion of Limbic System (Visceral Brain)." Electroencephalography and Clinical Neurophysiology 4:407-418.

MacLean, Paul D. 1970. "The Triune Brain, Emotion, and Scientific Bias." In The Neurosciences: Second Study Program, editor-in-chief F.O. Schmitt, 336-349. New York: The Rockefeller University Press.

MacLean, Paul D. 1977. "An Evolutionary Approach to Brain Research on Prosematic (Nonverbal) Behavior." In Reproductive Behavior and Evolution, ed. by J.R. Rosenblatt and B. Komisarus, 137-164. New York: Plenum Publishing Co.

MacLean, Paul D. 1978. "A Mind of Three Minds: Educating The Triune Brain." In Education and The Brain: The Seventy-seventh Yearbook of the National Society for the Study of Education. Part II, ed. by Jeanne S. Chall and Allan F. Mirsky, 308-342. Chicago: The University of Chicago Press.

MacLean, Paul D. 1982. "The Co-evolution of the Brain and Family." In Anthroquess, the L.S.B. Leakey Foundation News 24:1, 14-15. The L.S.B. Leakey Foundation: Pasadena, CA.

MacLean, Paul D. 1983. "Brain Roots of The Will-to-Power." Zygon: Journal of Religion and Science Vol. 18, No.4 (December):359-374.

MacLean, Paul D. 1985a. "Brain Evolution Relating to Family, Play and the Separation Call." Archives of General Psychiatry Vol. 42, April:405-417.

MacLean, Paul D. 1985b. "Evolutionary Psychiatry and the Triune Brain." Psychological Medicine 15:219-221.

Macquarrie, John. [1984] 1987. In Search of Deity: An Essay in Dialectical Theism. New York: The Crossroad Publishing Company.

Magoulias, Harry J. 1970. Byzantine Christianity: Emperor, Church, and the West. Chicago: Rand McNally & Company.

Mâle, Emile. [1913. 1958] 1972. The Gothic Image: Religious Art in France of the Thirteenth Century. Trans. by Dora Mussey. New York: Icon Editions, Harper & Row, Publishers.

Mandell, Arnold J. 1980. "Toward A Psychobiology of Transcendence: God in the Brain." In Psychobiology of Consciousness, eds. J.M.Davidson and R.J.Davidson, 379-464. New York: Plenum Press.

Martin, M.K. and B. Voohries. 1975. Female of the Species. New York: Columbia University Press.

Mathews, Thomas F. 1984. "Psychological Dimensions in the Art of Eastern Christendom." In Art and Religion: Faith, Form, and Reform. Paine Lectures in Religion, ed. by Osmund Overby. University of Missouri-Columbia.

McCoy, Kathleen. 1988. "5 Sex Secrets Women Wish Their Husbands Knew." Readers Digest, January, 91-94.

McFague, Sallie. 1975. Speaking in Parables: A Study in Metaphor and Theology. Philadelphia: Fortress Press.

McFague, Sallie. 1982. metaphorical theology: Models of God In Religious Language. Philadelphia: Fortress Press.

McFague, Sallie. 1987. Models of God: Theology for an Ecological, Nuclear Age. Philadelphia: Fortress Press.

McGlone, Jeannette. 1980. "Sex Differences in Human Brain Asymmetry: A Critical Survey." The Behavioral and Brain Sciences, 3:215-263.

McGuinnes, Diane and Karl Pribram. 1980. "Emotion and Motivation in Attention." In The Brain and Psychology, ed. by M.C. Wittrock. New York: Academic Press.

Meland, Bernard S., ed. 1969. The Future of Empirical Theology. Chicago: The University of Chicago Press.

Mendenhall, George E. 1955. "Law and Covenant in Israel and the Ancient Near East." The Biblical Colloquium. Pittsburgh.

Miller, Jean Baker. [1976] 1986. A New Psychology of Women. Boston: Beacon Press.

Milner, Brenda. 1962. "Laterality Affects in Audition." In Inter-Hemispheric Relations and Cerebral Dominance, ed. by V.B. Mountcastle. Baltimore: The John Hopkins Press.

Minsky, Marvin. [1985] 1986. The Society of Mind. New York: Simon and Schuster.

Moltmann, Jurgen. 1967. Theology of Hope. London: SCM Press Ltd.

Mondin, Battista. [1963] 1968. The Principle of Analogy in Protestant and Catholic Theology. Second revised ed. The Hague: Martinus Nijhoff.

Mountcastle, Vernon B. 1976. "The World Around Us: Neural Command Functions for Selective Attention." Neurosciences Research Program Bulletin Vol. 14, Supplement(April).

Myers, Jay J. 1984. "Right Hemisphere Language: Science or Fiction?" American Psychologist 39 (March):315-320.

Nathan, Peter. 1969. The Nervous System. Baltimore: Penguin Books, Inc.

Neisser, Urich. 1976. Cognition and Reality. San Francisco: W.H.Freeman and Company.

Nelson, David. 1987. Personal communication.

Nichols, Michael P. 1987. The Self in the System: Expanding the Limits of Family Therapy. New York: Brunner/Mazel Publishers.

Ornstein, Robert E. [1972, 1977] 1986. The Psychology of Consciousness. Completely revised and updated. New York: Penguin Books.

Ornstein, Robert E., ed. 1973. The Nature of Human Consciousness: A Book of Readings. San Francisco: W.H.Freeman and Company.

Ornstein, Robert. 1986. Multimind: A New Way of Looking at Human Behavior. Boston: Houghton Mifflin Company.

Ornstein, Robert and David **Sobel.** 1987. The Healing Brain: Breakthrough Discoveries About How the Brain Keeps Us Healthy. New York: A Touchstone Book.

Oscar-Berman, Marlene, Sheila **Blumstein,** and David **De Cosa.** 1976. "Iconic Recognition of Musical Symbols in the Lateral Visual Fields," Cortex 12, No.2 (September):241-248.

Panofsky, Erwin. 1957. Gothic Architecture and Scholasticism. New York: Meridian Books.

Patton, John and Brian H. **Childs.** 1988. Christian Marriage and Family: Caring for Our Generations. Nashville, TN: Abingdon.

Penfield, Wilder. 1975. The Mystery of the Mind: A Critical Study of Consciousness and the Human Brain. Princeton, NJ: Princeton University Press.

Perecman, Ellen, ed. 1984. Cognitive Processing in the Right Hemisphere. New York: Academic Press, Inc.

Perkins, D.N. 1981. The Mind's Best Work. Cambridge, MA: Harvard University Press.

Pierce, James David. 1986. A Multidimensional Scaling of The Cognitive Dimensions Used By Seminary Students in Their Perception of Biblical Material. Unpublished Dissertation. Evanston, IL: Northwestern University.

Polanyi, Michael. [1959] 1964. Personal Knowledge: Toward A Post-critical Philosophy. New York: Harper Torchbook.

Polanyi, Michael. 1966. The Tacit Dimension. New York: Doubleday.

Polanyi, Michael. 1968. "Logic and Psychology." American Psychologist, January, 27-43.

Prak, Liels Luning. 1968. The Language of Architecture: A Contribution to Architectural Theory. The Netherlands: Moutin & Co.

Pribram, Karl. 1985. "What The Fuss Is All About." In The Holographic Paradigm, ed. by Ken Wilber, 27-34. Boston: New Science Library/Shambhala.

Pribram, Karl. 1986. "The Cognitive Revolution and Mind/Brain Issues." American Psychologist Vol. 41, No. 5 (May):507-520.

Price, C.P. 1986. Virginia Seminary Journal (July):39.

Pritchard, James B., ed. 1969. Ancient Near Eastern Texts Relating to the Old Testament. Third edition with supplement. Princeton, NJ: Princeton University Press.

Procopius. [1940] 1961. Buildings, Volume VIII. Trans. by H.B.Dewing. The Loeb Classical Library. Cambridge, MA: Harvard University Press.

Rauschenbusch, Walter. 1909. Prayers of the Social Awakening. Boston: The Pilgrim Press.

Rauschenbusch, Walter. 1912. Christianity and the Social Crisis. New York: Association Press.

Rauschenbusch, Walter. 1919. A Theology for the Social Gospel. New York: The Macmillan Company.

Restak, Richard M. 1979. The Brain: The Last Frontier. New York: Warner Books.

Richardson, Alan and John **Bowden.** 1983. The Westminster Dictionary of Christian Theology. Phildelphia: The Westminster Press.

Ricoeur, Paul. 1978. "Manifestation and Proclamation." The Journal of the Blaisdell Institute 12 (Winter):13-35.

Robinson, John A.T. 1967. Exploration Into God. London: SCM Press Ltd.

Rosch, Eleanor. 1978. "Principles of Categorization." In Cognition and Categorization, ed. by Eleanor Rosch and Barbara B. Lloyd, 27-48. Hillsdale, NJ: Lawrence Erlbaum Associates.

Rosch, Eleanor and Barbara B. **Lloyd,** ed., 1978. Cognition and Categorization. Hillsdale, NJ: Lawrence Erlbaum Associates.

Rose, Hilary. [1983] 1987. "Hand, Brain, and Heart: A Feminist Epistemology for the Natural Sciences." In Sex and Scientific Inquiry, ed. by Sandra Harding and Jean F. O'Barr, 265-282. Chicago: The University of Chicago Press.

Rosenfeld, Anne H. 1985. "Music, The Beautiful Disturber." Psychology Today (Dec.):48-51,55.

Ross, Virginia. 1986. "The Transcendent Function of The Bilateral Brain." Zygon: Journal of Religion and Science Vol.21, No.2 (June):233-248.

Rossi, Ernest Lawrence. 1986. The Psychobiology of Mind-Body Healing. New Concepts of Therapeutic Hypnosis. New York: W.W. Norton & Company, Inc.

Rotenberg, Mordechai. 1986. "Hasidic Contradiction: A Model for Interhemispheric Dialogue." Zygon: Journal of Religion and Science Vol.21, No.2 (June):201-217.

Ruether, Rosemary Radford. 1983. Sexism and God-Talk: Toward a Feminist Theology. Boston: Beacon Press.

Rumelhart, David E., James L. **McClelland,** and the PDP Research Group. [1986] 1987. Explorations in the Microstructure of Cognition. Computational Models of Cognition and Perception. Vol. 1. Foundations, Vol. 2. Psychological and Biological Models. Cambridge, MA: MIT Press. A Bradford Book.

Russell, Jeffrey Burton. 1968. A History of Medieval Christianity: Prophecy and Order. New York: Thomas Y. Crowell Company.

Sachs, Oliver. [1984] 1987a. A Leg To Stand On. New York: Harper & Row.

Sachs, Oliver. [1970, 1981, 1983, 1984, 1985] 1987b. The Man Who Mistook His Wife for a Hat and Other Clinical Tales. New York: Harper & Row.

Samuels, Mike and Nancy **Samuels.** 1975. Seeing With The Mind's Eye: The History, Techniques and Uses of Visualization. New York: A Random House Bookworks Book.

Sanders, James A. 1987a. From Sacred Story to Sacred Text: Canon as Paradigm. Philadelphia: Fortress Press.

Sanders, James A. 1987b. The Challenge of Fundamentalism: One God and World Peace. Mimeographed lecture.

Schachtel, Ernest G. 1966. Experiential Foundations of Rorschach's Test. New York: Basic Books, Inc.

Schleiermacher, Frederick. 1958. On Religion: Speeches to Its Cultural Despisers. New York: Harper.

Selye, H. 1976. The Stress of Life. New York: McGraw-Hill.

Shah, Idries. [1964, 1969] 1971. The Sufis. London: Jonathan Cape.

Shah, Idries. [1978] 1981. Learning How To Learn: Psychology and Spirituality in the Sufi Way. Introduction by Doris Lessing. San Francisco: Harper & Row, Publishers.

Showalter, Elaine. 1987. "Medicine, Mind, and The Double Brain," by Anne Harrington, New York Times, Book Review, October 11.

Siegel, Bernie S. 1986. Love Medicine & Miracles: Lessons Learned About Self-Healing from a Surgeon's Experience with Exceptional Patients. New York: Harper & Row.

Simson, Otto von. [1956] 1974. The Gothic Cathedral: Origins of Gothic Architecture and the Medieval Concept of Order. Princeton, NJ: Princeton University Press, Bollingen Series XLVIII.

Skinner, James E. 1987. "How the Head Rules the Heart." In Life-Threatening Arrhythmias During Ischemia and Infraction," ed. by D. Hearse, A. Manning, and M. Janse, 135-151. New York: Raven Press.

Snyder, Solomon H. 1974. Madness and The Brain. New York: McGraw-Hill Book Company.

Somer, Robert. 1978. The Mind's Eye: Imagery in Everyday Life. New York: Delta.

Song, Choan-Seng. 1979. Third-eye Theology: Theology in Formation in Asian Settings. Maryknoll, NY: Orbis Books.

Southern, R.W. [1970] 1979. Western Society and The Churches in The Middle Ages. Baltimore: Penguin Books.

Sovik, E.A. 1973. Architecture For Worship. Minneapolis: Augsburg Publishing House.

Sperry, Roger W. 1968. "Hemisphere Deconnection and Unity in Conscious Awareness." American Psychologist 23:723-733.

Sperry, R.W. 1977. "Bridging Science and Values: A Unifying View of Mind and Brain." American Psychologist (April):237-245.

Sperry, Roger. 1982a. "Some Effects of Disconnecting the Cerebral Hemispheres." Science 24 (September) vol.217:1223-1226.

Sperry, R.W. 1982b. Science and Moral Priority: Merging Mind, Brain, and Human Values. New York: Columbia University Press.

Springer, Sally P. and Georg **Deutsch.** [1981] 1985. Left Brain, Right Brain. Rev. ed. New York: W.H. Freeman and Company.

Stinchcombe, Barbara. 1988. Personal conversation and correspondence about "The Brain and Belief." April-June.

Sullivan, Harry Stark. 1953. The Interpersonal Theory of Psychiatry. New York: W.W. Norton.

Sze, Mai-mai. [1956] 1959. The Way of Chinese Painting: Its Ideas and Technique. With selections from the Seventeenth century Mustard Seed Garden Manual of Painting. New York: Vintage Books.

Tanguay, Peter E. 1985. "Implications of Hemispheric Specialization for Psychiatry." In The Dual Brain: Hemispheric Specialization in Humans, ed. by D. Frank Benson and Eran Zaidel, 375-384. New York: The Guilford Press.

Taylor, Gordon Rattray. 1979. The Natural History of the Mind. New York: E.P.Dutton.

TenHouten, Warren D. 1985. "Cerebral-Lateralization Theory and The Sociology of Knowledge." In The Dual Brain: Hemispheric Specialization in Humans, ed. by D. Frank Benson and Eran Zaidel, 341-358. New York: The Guilford Press.

Terrace, H.S. 1985. "In the Beginning Was the 'Name.'" American Psychologist Vol. 40, No. 9 (September): 1011-1028.

The East. 1975. December, xi 10: 8-9.

Throcmorton, G.H. 1962. "Geneology (Christ)." In The Interpreter's Dictionary of The Bible: E-J, ed. George A. Buttrick, 365-366. New York: Abingdon Press.

Tillich, Paul. 1951. Systematic Theology. Vol. 1. Chicago: The University of Chicago Press.

Tillich, Paul. 1952. The Courage To Be. New Haven: Yale University Press.

Tillich, Paul. 1959. Theology of Culture, ed. by Robert C. Kimball. New York: Oxford University Press.

Tillich, Paul. 1968. A History of Christian Thought. Ed. by Carl E. Braaten. London: SCM Press Ltd.

Tillich, Paul. 1987. On Art and Architecture, ed. and with an Intro. by John Dillenberger, in collaboration with Jane Dillenberger. New York: Crossroads.

Tracy, David. 1981. The Analogical Imagination: Christian Theology and The Culture of Pluralism. Chicago: The University of Chicago Press.

Tracy, David. 1983. "The Analogical Imagination in Catholic Theology." In Talking About God: Doing Theology in the Context of Modern Pluralism, ed. David Tracy and John B. Cobb, Jr., intro David R. Mason, New York: The Seabury Press.

Trevarthen, Colwyn. 1986. "Brain Sciences and the Human Spirit." <u>Zygon: Journal of Religion and Science</u> Vol. 21, No.2 (June):161-200.

Troeger, Thomas H. 1980. <u>Rage, Reflect, Rejoice</u>. Philadelphia: Westminster Press.

Tucker, D.M. 1981. "Lateral Brain Function, Emotion and Conceptualization." <u>Psychological Bulletin</u> Vol. 89:19-46.

Turner, Victor. 1983. "Body, Brain and Culture." <u>Zygon: Journal of Religion and Science</u> Vol. 18, No.3 (September):221-245.

Ullman, Montague & Nan **Zimmerman.** [1979] 1980. <u>Working With Dreams</u>. New York: A Dell/Eleanor Friede Book.

Ullmann, Walter. 1966. <u>The Individual and Society in The Middle Ages</u>. Baltimore: The John Hopkins Press.

Underhill, Evelyn. [1911] 1961. <u>Mysticism</u>. New York: Dutton.

Vawter, Bruce. 1977. <u>On Genesis</u>. Garden City, NY: Doubleday & Company, Inc.

von Rod, Gerhard. 1961. <u>Genesis: A Commentary</u>. Translated by J.H. Marks. Philadelphia: The Westminster Press.

von Rod, Gerhard [1965] 1966. <u>The Problem of the Hexateuch and Other Essays</u>. Trans. by E.W. Truman Dicken, with an intro. by Norman W. Proteus. Edinburgh: Oliver and Boyd.

Waber, D.P. 1976. "Sex differences in cognition: a function of maturation rate?" Science, May: 572-573.

Waber, D.P. 1979. "Cognitive Abilities and Sex-related Variations." In Sex-related Differences in Cognitive Functioning: Developmental Issues, ed. by H.A. Wittig and A.C. Peterson. San Francisco: Academic Press.

Watzlawick, Paul. 1978. The Language of Change: Elements of Therapeutic Communication. New York: Basic Books, Inc.

Werner, E. 1962. "Music." In The Interpreter's Dictionary of The Bible: K-Q, ed. by George A. Buttrick, 457-469. New York: Abingdon Press.

Westerhoff, John W. 1979. "Contemporary Spirituality: Revelation, Myth and Ritual." In Aesthetic Dimensions of Religious Education, ed. by Gloria Durka & Joanmarie Smith, 13-27. New York: Paulist Press.

Westerman, Claus. [1971] 1974. Creation. Trans. by John J. Scullion, S.J. Philadelphia: Fortress Press.

Wilber, Ken, ed. 1985. The Holographic Paradigm and other Paradoxes: Exploring the Leading Edges of Science. Boston: New Science Library/Shambhala.

Wilke, John Thomas. 1981. A Neuro-Psychological Model of Knowing. Washington, D.C.: University Press of America.

Williams, Linda V. 1983. Teaching for the Two-Sided Brain. Englewood Cliffs, NJ: Prentice-Hall.

Williams, Roger. 1956. Biochemical Individuality: The Basis for the Genetotrophic Concept. New York: Wiley.

Winson, Jonathan. [1985] 1986. Brain & Psyche: The Biology of the Unconscious. New York: Vintage Books.

Witkin, H.A. and D.R. **Goodenough.** 1981. Cognitive Styles: Essence and Origins Field Dependence and Field Independence. New York: International Universities Press, Inc., Psychological Issues Monograph 51.

Wittig, H.A. and A.C. **Peterson,** eds. 1979. Sex-related Differences in Cognitive Functioning: Developmental Issues. San Francisco: Academic Press.

Wittrock, M.C., ed. 1980. The Brain and Psychology. New York: Academic Press.

Wolff, Hans Walter. 1974. Anthropology of the Old Testament. Philadelphia: Fortress Press.

Wonder, Jacquelyn and Priscilla **Donovan.** 1984. Whole-Brain Thinking: Working From Both Sides of the Brain to Achieve Peak Job Performance. New York: Ballantine Books.

Wong, Tony M. 1984. "One Brain's Response: A Reaction to Ashbrook's Juxtaposing the Brain and Belief." Journal of Psychology and Theology Vol. 12, No 3:208-210.

Young, Henry. 1987. "The Characteristics of Process Theology." Lectures, August 18-20, 25-27. Retreat Center, Notre Dame, IN.

Zaidel, Eran. 1985. "Implications: Introduction." In The Dual Brain: Hemispheric Specialization in Humans, ed. by D. Frank Benson and Eran Zaidel, 307-318. New York: The Guilford Press.

Zdenek, Marilee. 1983. The Right-Brain Experience: An Intimate Program to Free the Powers of Your Imagination. New York: Mc-Graw-Hill Book Company.

Zeig, Jeffrey K., ed. 1980. A Teaching Seminar With Milton H. Erickson, M.D. With commentary. New York: Brunner/Mazel, Publishers.

Zevi, Bruno. 1957. Architecture As Space: How to Look at Architecture. Trans. by Milton Gendel and ed. by Joseph A. Barry. New York: Horizon Press.

INDEX OF NAMES

INDEX OF SUBJECTS

INDEX OF SCRIPTURE